DISABILITY, OBESITY AND AGEING

The Cultural Politics of Media and Popular Culture

Series editor:
C. Richard King
Washington State University, USA

Dedicated to a renewed engagement with culture, this series fosters critical, contextual analyses and cross-disciplinary examinations of popular culture as a site of cultural politics. It welcomes theoretically grounded and critically engaged accounts of the politics of contemporary popular culture and the popular dimensions of cultural politics. Without being aligned to a specific theoretical or methodological approach, *The Cultural Politics of Media and Popular Culture* publishes monographs and edited collections that promote dialogues on central subjects, such as representation, identity, power, consumption, citizenship, desire and difference.

Offering approachable and insightful analyses that complicate race, class, gender, sexuality, (dis)ability and nation across various sites of production and consumption, including film, television, music, advertising, sport, fashion, food, youth, subcultures and new media, *The Cultural Politics of Media and Popular Culture* welcomes work that explores the importance of text, context and subtext as these relate to the ways in which popular culture works alongside hegemony.

Also available in this series:

Media and the Rhetoric of Body Perfection
Cosmetic Surgery, Weight Loss and Beauty in Popular Culture
Deborah Harris-Moore
ISBN: 978-1-4094-6944-5

Disability, Obesity and Ageing

Popular Media Identifications

DEBBIE RODAN
Edith Cowan University, Australia

KATIE ELLIS
Curtin University, Australia

PIA LEBECK
Murdoch University, Australia

Routledge
Taylor & Francis Group
LONDON AND NEW YORK

First published 2014 by Ashgate Publishing

Published 2016 by Routledge
2 Park Square, Milton Park, Abingdon, Oxfordshire OX14
711 Third Avenue, New York, NY 10017, USA

First issued in paperback 2016

Routledge is an imprint of the Taylor & Francis Group, an informa business

British Library Cataloguing in Publication Data
A catalogue record for this book is available from the British Library

The Library of Congress has cataloged the printed edition as follows:
Rodan, Debbie.
Disability, obesity and ageing : popular media identifications / by Debbie Rodan, Katie Ellis and Pia Lebeck.
pages cm. – (The cultural politics of media and popular culture)
Includes bibliographical references and index.
ISBN 978-1-4094-4051-2 (hardback)
1. Identity (Psychology) and mass media.
2. People with disabilities in mass media. 3. Obesity in mass media. 4. Older people in mass media. I. Ellis, Katie, 1978- II. Lebeck, Pia. III. Title.
P96.I34R63 2014
302.2301'9–dc23

2013026900

ISBN 13: 978-1-138-25459-6 (pbk)
ISBN 13: 978-1-4094-4051-2 (hbk)

Contents

Acknowledgements

The impetus for this book came from material used by Edith Cowan University undergraduate, masters-by-coursework, and masters of communication students in the unit MST3151/4151 *Media and Identity* across a number of years. We thank these students for their insights and enthusiasm; each teaching iteration offered us something more to think about and reinforced to us that disability, obesity and ageing really were popular media identifications.

Disability, Obesity and Ageing was made possible by several generous individuals and institutions and we thank them for their support and encouragement. We are grateful to the Centre for Research in Entertainment, Arts, Technology, Education and Communications (CREATEC) and Edith Cowan University for generous financial support and sabbatical leave (for Debbie). We want to express our appreciation to Maureen Lebeck, Ceri Ceriwyn, John Hall, Christine Brewer, Amanda Ellis and Carleen Ellis for their time in reading, preparing, formatting and proofreading the manuscript. Thank-you to Leanne Ellis and Kathryn Trees, in particular for their encouragement and unstinting support.

Debbie and Pia would like to thank their colleagues Rod Giblett, Jane Mummery and Carolyn Abbs who kindly shared their experience with us about writing. Their inspiration and thoughtful words of encouragement enabled us to see the project to the end. David Smyth provided home-based technical support by ensuring television recording and computer equipment as well as software programs were optimized to keep the writing on track.

Katie would like to thank her colleagues and students in the school of Media Communication and Culture at Murdoch University where she was based for the majority of the project. In particular Mick Broderick, Kai-Ti Kao, Felicity Newman and students in MCC235 for their crucial support, encouragement and insightful conversations about popular culture and television. She is grateful also to Gerard Goggin, Tara Brabazon, Beth Haller, Petra Kuppers and Mike Kent for their inspirational work, guidance and insightful questions. She wishes to thank her family – Chris and Stella – for their unwavering support across the duration of this project. Also to Fay Davidson for her abiding interest, personally and professionally. Finally thanks to colleagues in the department of Internet Studies at Curtin University where the book was finished.

At Ashgate Publishing Neil Jordan who saw the potential of this book, and helped us shape it and to C. Richard King for inviting us to be part of

The Cultural Politics of Media and Popular Culture series. Thanks also go to the anonymous reviewers, all of whom gave such helpful feedback.

Parts of Chapter 6 were first published as "Remaking the Obese 'Self' in The Biggest Loser: Couples (Australia)" in Proceedings of the Australian and New Zealand Communication Association on Media Democracy and Change Conference (2010) (see http://www.canberra.edu.au/anzca2010/conference-proceedings). We thank the editor Kerry McCallum for her support, encouragement and permission to republish here.

PART I
Television as a Social Experience

Chapter 1
Introduction: Renegotiating Disability, Obesity and Ageing

In 2012, *Betty White's Off Their Rockers* aired on Betty White's ninetieth birthday. The programme's official website claimed the candid-camera-style prank show would take 'senior stereotypes and [blow] them out of the water with a cast of sassy septuagenarians who are hip, sexy and ready to party'. Online reviewer meltinzone (2012) engages with the process of his own ageing when he expresses his admiration for the new show and elderly television personality, Betty White:

> As a 24 year old guy with an awesome sense of humour, well Betty White has always appealed to me […] I was half expecting the show to be about old people 'off their rockers' and to my delight it's about old people pranking the more youthful, though it appears no one is too old to be pranked.

This post negotiates the meaning of old age by simultaneously reinforcing and undermining its quantification. meltinzone disidentifies with White and her elderly companions by claiming he is relatively young. His minimization of his ageing identity is further strengthened by his characterization of being 'off one's rocker' as a form of age-induced decline he would prefer not to see on television. At the same time, meltinzone's suggestion that humour is a means of transcending categories of age recognizes ageing as an ongoing process.

Producer Chuck Lorre introduced an innovative new television programme, *Mike & Molly* in 2010. In this romantic situation comedy, created by Mark Roberts, plus-sized or fat actors took on leading roles to depict the struggle larger people have in finding love. Lorre believed it was time to deal with a theme about 'people who feel as if they have lost hope at having a meaningful relationship' (cited in Idato, 2011, p. 201). Yet several online audience members discussing *Mike & Molly* implicitly pointed to the power of the television text to objectify the obese body by critiquing particular storylines and costume choices. Discussions on the *Television Without Pity* forum reveal these audiences are familiar with the situation comedy genre, and its rather narrow repertoire of representations. The viewers criticized scriptwriters for sticking with the generic formula of situation comedies:

> Am I alone in feeling that Molly's just being given the standard Bitch Girlfriend script? I had a longer post, but essentially it was the growing disappointment talking (Actionmage, 2011).

A winemaker and businessman with cerebral palsy auditioned for the 2009 season of *MasterChef* Australia. John Hughes progressed through to the top 40 but then willingly entered the elimination round, which would decide the top 24 contestants, by refusing to present a dish. Part way through the challenge he approached guest judge and high profile cookbook author Maggie Beer and told her he was struggling with the time constraints. Prior to the challenge he had been offered extra time to read and interpret the recipes to compensate for the effects of his impairment. However, he had refused this offer, not wanting to be 'treated differently' (McCormick, 2011, p. 13). Although he had already made the fatal mistake of using wet flour instead of dry in his cake, Maggie simply encouraged him to start again.

John's inability to complete the dish due to time limits demonstrates that despite the rhetoric of much disability representation, sometimes people with disability require alternative arrangements – such as extra time – to complete tasks to the same standard as non-disabled people. Yet John was touted, within the programme and in the wider media, as inspirational for trying and then refusing to serve up a dish he considered substandard. However, this construction was recognized and critiqued online:

> I was touched by John last night, and totally appalled at channel 10. The selection criteria used to select the initial pool of contestants is not based on skill, but rather personality, looks, or how well the person will appeal to the public, and thus have a positive effect on ratings. I doubt Johns skills would ever come into question in this game show, but when he said to Maggie Beer halfway through that he was struggling with time, and that he could do it, but to his own time, I could instantly see the plan from Channel 10. He is not there because of his skill but because of his Cerebral Palsy. It will be used by Channel ten to milk the emotions of every viewer as much as possible, and John deserves far better than that. I am certain that John would want to be looked on as the cook who tried his best, rather than 'that poor disabled guy' yet it is that 'poor disabled guy' image that Channel 10 want to garner for him (TheLoneOutsider, 2011).

These are a few vignettes to illustrate the increasing visibility of disability, obesity and ageing on popular television and the ways audiences are negotiating the meanings presented to them using online platforms. This book evaluates depictions – as well as online audience reactions to them – of disability, obesity and ageing in a range of televisual genres. The focus is on television programmes and accompanying websites because television is still the most watched medium and increasingly involves a corresponding and simultaneous online engagement.

Whereas limited repertoires are presented on television, new media forums offer new models for constructing and circulating identities. Online discussions of television images constitute a culturally significant, ongoing and open-ended body of work, a text through which we can explore social attitudes. These discussions are a vital resource for considering public representations of disability, obesity and ageing in a culture that is both saturated with visual images and highly conscious of the normative body.

Disability, obesity and ageing are subject to a social disablement whereby social acceptance relies on the individual's willingness to adapt. Whereas in 1989 Diane Driedger (p. 1) described the social model of disability as 'the last civil rights movement', the more recent emergence of the seniors and so-called fat acceptance movements suggests the concepts of civil rights and social disablement, now advanced in disability studies, can be applied to other marginalized groups. The social model of disability argues people are disabled and disempowered, not by their bodies but by inflexible social practices and power imbalances which are based on a view that these bodies are inferior. Age and obesity are likewise subjected to similar disabling social attitudes. Following on from recent work which connects or groups disability, obesity and ageing as non-normative, problem or rejected bodies (Chivers & Markotić, 2010; Richardson, 2010; Wendell, 1996), we aim to further these scholarly conversations by expanding the insights, offered through understandings of social disablement, to ageing and obesity throughout this book.

Ideal Bodies and Representational Systems: Why Disability, Obesity and Ageing?

Much media and cultural studies analysis to date has focused on examining and articulating how the media depict gender, sexuality, race, and class; however, in this book we turn to an analysis of depictions of disability, obesity and ageing. These three categories are loosely connected as stigmatized identities. Television programmes typically depict these groups as abnormal or peripheral. However, the chapters that follow illustrate a new paradigm whereby characters who are disabled, ageing or obese occupy important narrative roles. Despite this increase in representation, disability, obesity and ageing continue to be rejected as abnormal bodies.

Television covers and represents disability, obesity and ageing within a similarly narrow range. For example, qualitative and quantitative studies report the portrayal of disability on television is inadequate and stereotypical (Cumberbatch & Negrine, 1992), whereas televisual portrayals of fat people perpetuate fat stigma (Himes & Thompson, 2007), and older people are subject to marginal roles on-screen (Donlon, Ashman, & Levy, 2005, p. 315). Although each identification is a dynamic and complex intersection between the body, the self and society, televisual images are often essentialized and narrowly framed.

We discuss a variety of programmes in this book and intentionally do not focus on any particular genre. This cross-genre approach – drama, situation comedies, reality television, documentary – reveals intertextual patterns of representation. Such an approach allows us to focus on the ubiquity of disability, obesity and ageing as a dominant thematic concern. Each programme we consider has rated well with audiences and was initially scheduled during primetime. Indeed, at the height of each programme's broadcast, they achieved what Lotz describes as water-cooler status (2007). We offer this variety of analysis to demonstrate the ongoing popularity of disability, obesity and ageing as televisual identifications, despite their socially spurned positions.

In addition, we discuss a variety of online platforms throughout this book, including both official and unofficial television forums. This relatively new media environment and practice of engaging with televisual texts has also facilitated the rise of online activist groups affiliated with disability, fat acceptance and seniors' social justice. This book interrogates the relationship between television, culture and social attitudes towards disability, obesity and ageing across a number of television and online texts.

Televisual representations continue to rely on prejudicial attitudes regarding acceptable bodies that circulate in the media and historical representations of disability, obesity and ageing. This book seeks to take into account this so called 'tacit body knowledges' (Murray, 2007, p. 370) and whether it applies in the current era of television overflow onto online texts. Several theorists have identified 'overflow' as a modern manifestation of Raymond Williams' famous concept of television 'flow' (Brooker, 2004; Gillan, 2011; Gray, 2008). Writing in 1974 Williams argued television networks held control over what viewers watched and offered a particular programming configuration where 'narrative, advertisements and promotions all intermixed' (Lotz, 2007, p. 34). This purported flow was structured to suit the broadcasters and usually reflected middle-class interests. Whereas Williams in his book *Television – Technology and Cultural Form*, (1974, p. 151) predicted flow would be disrupted by localized programming and participatory democracy, recent technological and social developments have brought about circular flow, where audiences remain engaged with the programme on various levels and mediums. People engage with this overflow to create meaningful contexts on blogs and television companion websites despite television's limited available cultural identities.

From Representation to Identification

The emergence of audience response websites, such as *Digital Spy*, *TV.com* and *Television Without Pity*, and other forms of audience online engagement represent a crucial moment in the study of television. These sites allow us to examine public interpretations about disability, obesity and ageing which have traditionally been relegated to the periphery of mainstream media attention. Historically, obesity, disability and ageing have been subject to discourses of exclusion that shore up boundaries of normality through 'binary processes of demarcation' (Johnson, 2008, p. 44). Throughout this book we approach both television programmes and online discussion as representative cultural texts regarding public attitudes about disability, obesity and ageing. We further approach this analysis from the perspective of identification or the way identity engages audience members during reception (Cohen, 2001, p. 261). According to Jonathan Cohen (p. 261), 'identification is an imaginative process through which an audience member assumes the identity, goals, and perspective of a character'. Sympathetic and intriguingly unsympathetic characters, as identification targets, increase audience involvement in a television text. Similarly, online forums also operate as identification targets, allowing us to see this phenomenon in process.

Online Spaces and the Politicization of Disability, Obesity and Ageing

Some disability bloggers believe online discussion represents a way forward for disability theorization and representation. These spaces include and influence the non-disabled population or those with disabilities unaware of the politicization of their identities:

> Readers comment that they have had no previous knowledge about or interest in disability, but having enjoyed what we've written about other issues or personal interests, and are learning almost by accident, becoming conscious of the environment, systems and behaviours which disable us. Only on personal blogs have I read accounts of the big ideas, such as the Social Model of Disability, written in a light-hearted, easily digestible way. It is to such blog-entries that I now direct people when I am trying to explain these things, as opposed to traditional academic resources (The Goldfish, 2007).

User generated content also holds an important position within the experience of viewing and reviewing television, especially in the formation of communities of interest. Bronwyn Williams (2009) considers this relationship and posits that the interactive nature of new media has had an effect on the study of popular culture such as television – people with disparate interests are brought together and assist one another in the process of making meaning.

As The Goldfish (2007) argues, people are brought together in online discourse, learning complex ideas about social disablement and impairment effects, 'almost by accident'.

Much of the online discussion we explore in this book demonstrates that binary thinking continues to inform people's attitudes towards disability, obesity, and ageing. For example, discussions surrounding obese bodies as unproductive circulate in online forums and ageing is often considered in the binary context of vigour/slowness. We seek to expose implicit commonsense but disabling understandings about disability, obesity and ageing and the elaborate social hierarchies that create and support them. The cultural stigma imposed on disability, obesity and ageing is the result of complex histories and relations of power – they take in multiple discourses.

Visions of the World: Discourse and Symbolic Power

Disability, obesity and ageing are unquantifiable states of being. Their meanings have changed across time and are context specific. Everyone becomes old, or at least older, with at least 25 per cent of people disabled, overweight or both. What the categories of disability, obesity and ageing represent is a lack of control of the body. As such, these representations become discomforting to many individuals who prefer to believe they are in total control of their bodies and, by extension, themselves.

Disability, obesity and ageing are negated forms of subjectivity and undesirable states of embodiment. Reducing individual subjects to their bodies is a form of narrative strategy that reflects a wider culture of denial and deferral. Denying the voices of characters that are disabled, obese or old parallels the refuted construction of their bodies. The naturalized repudiation of these non-normative bodies is signified by the (continuing) popularity of narratives about reforming, erasing, reclaiming, perfecting and overcoming body limitations and the various forms of stigma with which they are associated. Such constructions normalize the assumption that the disabled, old and obese should defer to those who are non-disabled, slim and young.

Televisual discourse mediates reality through the way it 'reflects and constructs particular values and beliefs about different aspects of "reality"' (Lorenzo-Dus, 2009, p. 189). Throughout the book a discourse analysis will be used to illustrate the manner in which the media tries to qualify or impose identifications as facts, without qualification. Discursive practices objectify and subjugate those deemed disabled, obese and old, by creating the view that these subject positions are not desirable. Linda Graham observes that as a result of 'processes of objectification, individuals not only come to occupy *spaces* in the social hierarchy but, through their continual subjugation, come to know and accept their *place*' (2011, p. 672). We use Foucault's concept of discourse throughout this book to explore how contemporary media practices position the disabled, old and obese, while also functioning as sites of contestation and potential release.

Television, as a mass media, is seen to have the power to influence attitudes and beliefs about political and social issues, particular groups and specific events (Finkelstein, 2012). For example, a Glasgow Group study into the representation of people with mental illness found, despite positive professional interactions with people who had mental health conditions, respondents believed the media stereotype that people with mental health conditions are a violent threat (Philo, Secker, Platt, Hendersen, McLaughlin, & Burnside, 1994). Couldry (2002, p. 4) describes this as television's 'symbolic power'. For Bourdieu, symbolic power encourages people to see and 'believe' or transform their 'vision of the world' (Bourdieu, 1991, p. 170). Television's symbolic power can be seen in the narrow range of representations of disability, obesity and ageing and the ways these have influenced and entered public discourse about these groups. By drawing on a habitual way of speaking about disability (Barnes, 1992), obesity (Richardson, 2010) and ageing (Signorielli, 2004), television legitimizes already held beliefs to reinforce social reality for many people (see Bourdieu, p. 166). The repetition of certain imagery implies 'we' all collectively share this particular belief (Couldry, 2002, p. 4). Predictable and formulaic portrayals of people with disabilities and those who are obese, and old, reinforce the media's social authority to typecast particular groups. Viewers, like those in the Glasgow Group research, might think 'I know people who are not like that', yet still retain conventional beliefs about these identity categories which are depicted on television. By drawing on, reinforcing and circulating commonly held beliefs and stereotypes, television media plays a significant role in shoring up a media discourse about a particular group.

Although we argue disability, obesity and ageing are loosely connected by their televisual spurned position, and that they are all subject to social disablement, some clear deviations exist between these groups in terms of their research histories, televisual representation and online presence. Despite their relative status and differing research and social justice histories, these identity positions are connected by television's arbitrary attempts to quantify them. Televisual discourse constructs a clear divide between those who are disabled, old and obese, and those who are not.

Disability: An Undesirable Identity

Disability as a cultural category occupies an uncomfortable position in identity politics. Previously viewed only as a medical problem, with little relevance to cultural studies or the humanities broadly, disability has more recently been recognized as a social, cultural and political category. The social model of disability identifies disability can be environmental (such as inaccessible buildings, services, languages), organizational (inflexible practices, procedures and people), and attitudinal (prejudice, stereotypes and discrimination).

Disability has long been represented as an undesirable identity on television. It is used as a visual reference to denote evil or represented as an unspeakable tragedy that must be cured through inspirational personal qualities and medical intervention. There has been a significant increase of characters with disability on television, to the point where disability is now part of the Gay and Lesbian Alliance Against Defamation (GLAAD) exploration of whether series regular characters on US television exhibit sexual, racial, ethnic (and now disability), diversity. Their 2012–2013 study, however, noted only 0.6 per cent of characters had a disability (GLAAD, 2013, p. 15).

For Mitchell and Snyder (2000), critical analysis of these images of disability represents an engagement with disability culture without privileging a certain type of representation. They argue that critical analysis of these images and their interactions offer a way to identify the 'culture that *might be* rather than that which *is*' (Mitchell & Snyder, p. 45). This imagining of a culture that might be is taking place on online audience forums and popular culture blogs. Disability operates as a vehicle of meaning-making in narrative discourses, a so-called narrative prosthesis (cf. Mitchell & Snyder). For example, disability has been used as an aid to denote weakness or a loss of control. Obesity and ageing operate within narrative discourses in a similar way.

Obesity: A New Cultural Phenomenon

Supporting characters on-screen that are fat are often included for comedic purposes or used as a narrative prosthesis to add a dimension of characterization to slim main characters. The slim body is the norm on television, a body that is unrepresentative of the general population. Despite this history, there are now more oversized bodies on television than ever before. In effect, the number of fat bodies on television – often referred to as the obese body – is a new cultural phenomenon.

The ways in which the obese body is depicted fascinates both audiences and others in the public realm such as medical, science and health practitioners, and television programme makers. Thus, looking at how the fat body is portrayed – in particular, the way television media endeavours to essentialize what is an obese body – is a vital topic to research and analyse.

There has been a significant increase in the number of fat bodies in the makeover genre in particular. These makeover–lifestyle–health programmes construct the fat body as obese by offering contestants and participants limited roles.

Televisual media draws on medical and personal training discourse, which is inflected with cultural views about fitness and fatness, in its attempt to quantify the obese body. In many of these programmes, ordinary people are likely to be depicted in derisory ways, so producers can attract audiences and increase ratings (Turner, 2009, p. 69).

The obese body is a source of fascination for some audience members because it is different. For others, they identify with the obese body and feel empathy for those who are trying to lose weight. For another set, aspects of the programme are of interest such as insights into how people become obese, how to change established eating habits and how to change lifestyle patterns. For many, however, the obese body is seen as abnormal – a body 'out of control' (Wendell, 1996, p. 98).

Ageing: Mobilizing Economic Forces

Although television has not entirely neglected older people, research shows they have been consistently underrepresented and relegated to stereotypical and peripheral roles. Dramas and sitcoms have rarely featured narratives based on the lives of older characters, and older actors have tended to be cast in familiar, yet narrow roles. The tendency to marginalize and stereotype ageing characters on television has resulted in easily recognizable and reductive performances of older age. Television genres have reinforced this homogenizing impetus through particular representations of gender and ageing. For example, standard tropes such as the ageing matriarch in soaps and melodramas, and the accomplished, mature anchor man in current affairs and broadcast news, have set the agenda for television audiences' expectations about growing older. Importantly, these motifs are now the basis on which burgeoning images of older people on the small screen can be measured and discussed.

Current popular television reflects a changing social landscape of older age with a move from standard tropes to more diverse representations. The unprecedented visibility of older bodies mirrors the global demographics of population ageing. This trend parallels the present rise of contemporary television drama as a serious narrative form. Its episodic structure and extended treatment of time is conducive to themes of ageing and later life. In addition to drama, television presents an array of formats and programmes, with the capacity to reflect mature experience. Notable among these are reality makeover programmes such as *10 Years Younger in 10 Days* and *Hotter Than My Daughter*, each of which draws on the neo-liberal ethos of market forces, positing ageing as the focus of individual management and consumer choices. In this paradigm, ageing is predominantly a matter of mobilizing social and economic resources (Featherstone & Wernick, 1995).

It is clear that disability, obesity and ageing are essentialized on television and when taken together represent a thematic fascination regarding rejected bodies across several formats and genres. This thematic fascination has similarly been embraced by online audiences. Online forums are discursive spaces where audiences can create and respond to representations of cultural normativity through conversations about television programmes.

Overview

A key focus of the discussion in this book is the ways discourses function – how particular understandings about disability, obesity and ageing are validated and made to appear normal. Each of the programmes has their dominant discourse about disability, obesity and ageing which may differ or confer with online audience responses to the show. An investigation of competing discourses allows us to consider which discourse is given import and which are considered of lesser value and, as a consequence, lack influence. How online audiences interact with each other about the programmes is an integral part of televisual consumption. In this sense, the audience as consumers of online forums do not simply read the information and take it on board; they tend to also 'decode texts' (Condit cited in Richardson, 2007, p. 41).

The book is divided into two parts. We show how disability, obesity and ageing are pervasive issues. Part I comprises three chapters which consider *Television as a Social Experience* to establish connections between disability, obesity and ageing as well as the relevance of online audience activity and identification. Following this, Part II – *Identifications* – recognizes the specific research histories of each category to explore in depth case studies of disability, obesity and ageing as popular media identifications.

We begin Part I by exploring the historical meanings ascribed to disability, obesity and ageing as they have emerged through other modes of cultural production such as freak shows, medical pamphlets and literature in Chapter 2, *Tacit Knowledge: Cultural Representations of Disability, Obesity and Ageing*. Cultural texts provide both an insight into the social position of disability, obesity and ageing during the time in which they were made and offer a foundation on which to base televisual representations. Images of old, obese and/or disabled bodies have long been considered aesthetically challenging and unwatchable by the general public. Viewers may have found such images difficult to see because they did not have a readily accessible frame of reference to accommodate their reception and understanding.

Chapter 3, *A Marketplace of Ideas: Television as a Social Experience* examines the ways in which television is a potent medium for representing our identity categories of disability, obesity and ageing. Television affords people the opportunity to meet people outside their family, friendship and work circles – people they can only know about through images in the popular media. In addition, this chapter focuses on the ways televisual representations of disability, obesity and ageing are publicly debated online. We consider both social activist sites, initiated by disability, seniors, feminist and fat acceptance groups, and those that emerge around particular television programmes. We explore the common themes that materialize in online discussion of televisual representations of disability, obesity and ageing to examine how the media's symbolic power is being contested and or reinforced. We argue that through these discussions, online audiences introduce critiques and new ways of thinking about disability, obesity and ageing.

Chapter 4, *Audience Activity: Identification, Disidentification and Online Activity,* moves to an examination of the insight online discussion provide regarding the acceptance or rejection of disability, obesity and ageing as problem bodies. Our analysis is framed from the perspective of identification. For Cohen (2001), identifying with characters or participants occurs when audiences share the same characteristics, interests, affinities and experiences. We explore the ways television producers use stylistic techniques such as framing and music to encourage both identification and disidentification in terms of the types of discussion taking place in official and unofficial television forums. This online discussion allows us to consider the effects of the construction of the television text.

While illustrative case studies are used throughout Part I of the book, Part II *Identifications,* includes chapters which consider case studies of popular representations of disability, obesity and ageing in significant depth. We begin with disability in Chapter 5, *Disability Drama.* People with disability negotiate a complex identity that involves both physical difference and social stigma. When approached from an individual model, disability is something that a person must overcome, and the social restrictions are not addressed. Individualized images of disability feature in every television genre from news and current affairs to reality television and drama. This chapter explores the way online audiences negotiate what could be described as disabling televisual imagery by examining representations of disability in Season 2 of the critically acclaimed Australian television drama *Packed to the Rafters* along with online audience response to the portrayal. The American musical dramedy *Glee* is also analysed to illustrate the ways disability is used as a narrative prosthesis and the tendency of online disability activists to reject these portrayals.

Chapter 6, *Obesity Makeover: Rejecting the Obese Body,* turns to a discussion of the gradual increase of the obese body on television. This chapter's main focus is Season 4 of *The Biggest Loser* (Australia) – *The Biggest Loser: Couples* (2009). We provide an in-depth analysis of the series as well as the official online forum as an example of television overflow. One of the main claims made explicit in the programme is that thinner people are *happier* and *freer* than obese people.

Foucault's observations around disciplining bodies provide some insights into the common narratives used to construct fat characters on television. One of those techniques is to transform contestants' personhood so that they reject the obese body to become free. However, this claim to freedom does not account for the lack of freedom that results from the new regulations these contestants must embrace.

The media tries to quantify age, alongside disability and obesity. Chapter 7, *Ageing Transformations: Embracing the 'Young–Old' Body*, considers ageing as a popular media identification. Contemporary media images both reinforce negative perceptions of ageing and create communicative spaces for reflection and attitudinal change. Ageing is simultaneously defined, on the one hand, by burgeoning visual representations of older people and, on the other, by idealized images of youthfulness. In this context, ageing troubles representation at precisely the same time as the increasing visibility of older bodies familiarizes later life (Basting, 1998; Woodward, 1991). We focus on Season 1 of the Australian makeover reality series *10 Years Younger in 10 Days* and related websites and discussion forums, to argue a key challenge for contemporary media is to reconceptualize ageing as a productive process of change. This is especially so when popular televisual discourse constructs staying young as the responsibility of individuals.

This individualization of adaptation is a theme that unites disability, obesity and ageing. We're all likely to experience disablement at some point in our lives – especially if we survive into old age. As such we argue that all three identifications can be located within critical models of disability. The conclusion to the book – *Beyond the Water-cooler* – argues a critical understanding of disability, obesity and ageing allows us to appreciate how televisual representations are highly normative and influential for fundamental ideas of ourselves, our relationships with each other, what is normal, and how society is constructed. The televisual representations and online discussions analysed throughout the book also initiates a more in-depth understanding of diversity in televisual media, and what this might mean. In drawing parallels between disability, obesity and ageing it is not our intention to claim media representations are definitive or predominantly positive or negative. Instead, we suggest that in the contemporary media environment, disability, obesity and ageing are part of an ongoing process whereby meaning is actively and constantly engaged and (re)negotiated.

Chapter 2
Tacit Knowledge: Cultural Representations of Disability, Obesity and Ageing

> For many, both disabled and non-disabled people, the biggest obstacle to disabled people's meaningful inclusion into mainstream community life is negative public attitudes. These range from overt prejudice and hostility, condescension and pity to ignorance and indifference, and in these diverse ways they influence how we think about both ourselves and other people (Barnes, 1997, p. 3).

> Anything on television can frame and represent reality, but a key question for analysis should be: does this programme encourage me to seek out reality, or does it encourage me to replace reality with fiction and untruths, and to produce yet more 'thems' that can be contrasted to 'us'? (Gray, 2008, p. 121).

A number of writers consider that the individual's understanding of the contemporary world comes mainly from the modern media. From this perspective, the media provides entertainment, information and opinions about the world in which we live. As both Barnes and Gray note in the epigraphs to the chapter, media representations affect public attitudes, especially regarding marginalized groups such as people who are disabled, old and/or obese. According to Gray, television entertainment makes proclamations about what is normal and abnormal (2008 p. 157). He states that television continues old norms and relies on stereotypes that 'essentialize a group of people' (p. 111), including those who are disabled, obese or old. Susan Wendell (1996) agrees, arguing that their bodies transgress the cultural boundaries of normality because they are too distant from the ideal body. She adds that people are 'subjected to cultural pressure' and prone to feel ashamed of their body if it is too removed 'from the ideals' (p. 91). In twenty-first century Western society, the pressure to be young, fit and without physical impairment is especially keen on television and fosters 'a desire to gain/maintain control of our bodies' (p. 91). We believe this televisual ideal body – which is increasingly being conflated with the norm – has materialized through a long tradition of cultural representation.

Representations of and understandings about disability, obesity and ageing draw on a long, intertextual cultural history, and many of the verbal and visual signifiers used in earlier media are circulated and repurposed in twenty-first century televisual media and online forums. For example, D.H. Lawrence's use of an impotent, disabled man in *Lady Chatterley's Lover* to represent all that he thought was wrong with modern industrial society (Shakespeare, 1994, p. 285) draws on a problematic cultural history of the relationship between disability and masculinity. Hegemonic masculinity is predicated on the absence of impairment, therefore the presence of disability in cultural representations is easily recognized as a loss of masculinity.

This discursive link between masculinity and disability continues to provide the basis from which other representations, such as film and television, and even online discussion, can draw. Snyder and Mitchell (2006, p. 201) encourage disability theorists to engage in exhaustive textual analysis to uncover the way cultural beliefs about disability are reflected in visual and written materials. These discursive links, and disabling social attitudes, also evident in televisual representations of obese and ageing bodies, rely on internalized social statements which Samantha Murray (2007, p. 363) describes as 'tacit' knowledge.

The chapter begins with a discussion of representation and the ways disability, obesity and ageing have been considered unwatchable or peripheral, before moving on to specific discussions of historical representations of these identity categories. The focus is mainly on stereotypes of these groups and the ways in which they repeatedly emerge. In the last 40 years in particular, feminist media theorists have noted the importance of evaluating stereotypical images as a way to facilitate an awareness of alternatives. Using these insights, disability, fat and ageing studies theorists similarly interrogate stereotypes as a way to develop awareness, critical thinking and debunk disabling social attitudes. Our analysis builds on the trajectory of critical media analysis that has followed Tuchman's (1978) argument that a symbolic annihilation is evident in the limited roles for women in media representation. Tuchman's observation that women were omitted, trivialized and condemned by the media through the construction of specific social roles can be applied to representations of disability, obesity and ageing, albeit in a somewhat modified fashion.

After exploring the specific cultural histories of disability, obesity and ageing throughout the chapter, we finish with a discussion of the representational importance of online discussion as a relatively new text worthy of cultural analysis, especially with regard to representations of disability, obesity and ageing. Following the introduction of television companion websites in the late 1990s, media studies scholars began noting the importance of new media to both the experience and study of television (Livingstone, 1999). These mediated discussions both critique *and* draw on stereotypes and tacit knowledge. In addition to offering insight into the ways audiences negotiate televisual messages, these discussions are a form of representation themselves, influenced by culture and context. Certainly, watching television today is not what it used to be, even compared to only a few years ago. Although what constitutes television and the ways we watch it may have changed, the images we see and the way we respond to them and discuss them online are often uncannily familiar, drawing as they do on a long tradition of cultural representation.

Representation

According to Jen Webb, representations shape our experiences of the world (2009, p. 2). Using women as an example of the way critical analysis of representations can uncover 'embedded, underlying meanings of texts' (p. 1), Webb explains:

> How women are represented in film, for instance, can be seen to convey both the attitude of the film maker to women, and the general way women are viewed, understood, or 'known' in a particular context – the context in which the film was made and distributed. (p. 1)

Webb's argument that 'representation governs our experience of the world' (p. 4) echoes the sentiments expressed by both Barnes (1997) and Gray (2008) in the epigraphs to this chapter. Tom Shakespeare (1994) emphasizes the importance of representation to the social position of people with disability when he argues people with disability are subject to prejudice as a result of cultural representations, language and socialization. His observation that different mythologies surround different impairments invites an analysis of disability, obesity and ageing as problem bodies subject to prejudice. A consideration of tacit knowledge, cultural representation, language and socialization reveals the ways obesity and ageing have been subject to disabling social attitudes. Just as cultural texts rely on different prejudice and mythologies when representing autism, as opposed to hearing or vision impairment for example, representations of obesity and ageing draw on other social anxieties and internalized social statements.

As we discussed in the previous chapter, representations of disability, obesity and ageing are loosely connected via their histories of negation and subjugation. They have been subject to a symbolic annihilation (Tuchman, 1978, p. 8) through the media's promotion of stereotypes and strategies of exclusion. During the 1970s, Tuchman argued that media representation provided a limited trajectory for women. She surmised that women were represented in three ways in the media: first, women were omitted or absent from arenas outside the home such as the workplace (p. 29); second, when women did appear on television they were trivialized; and third when women appeared outside the role of mother and wife they were condemned.

Tuchman's framework has been applied to the critical analysis of a number of other socially constructed and marginalized groups to illustrate the ways the media devalues them. For example, critical analysis of race, sexual orientation and class are well established within media studies – critical disability, obesity and ageing studies are emerging through these traditions. Indeed, like women in Tuchman's 1978 study, we observe that people who are disabled, obese and old are omitted, trivialized and condemned on television. The majority of characters and participants on television are non-disabled, slim and young. When characters with disability, obesity or who are old are represented on television, they are often victimized, isolated or shown in supporting roles. Further, these characters are frequently condemned for failing to fit into society's conception of normality, a notion which is increasingly conflated with the ideal.

There is also a sense in which, until recently, images of bodies that were old, obese and/or disabled were 'unrepresentable' (Webb, 2009, pp. 4–5) because the public considered them aesthetically challenging and/or inappropriate; a 'normative formula' for regarding acceptable bodies dominates (Snyder & Mitchell, 2010, p. 193). Viewers may have found such images difficult to see because they did not have a readily accessible frame of reference to accommodate their reception and understanding.

On the Periphery

Commonly characters who are disabled, old or obese have been relegated to peripheral roles. Lloyd (2010) describes fat characters as 'carrying water for the svelte', and Barnes (1992) believes peripheral characters with disability encourage 'a lewd fascination' that draws on pre-existing social prejudice surrounding disability as a freak show. Similarly, several scholars have noted that the marginalization of older characters on primetime television is evidenced by their peripheral status (Healey & Ross, 2002; Signorielli, 2004). As Jake Harwood suggests, absent or peripheral characters offer a significant insight into who is valued in society:

> If we want to understand where a group stands in society, there are few better ways of getting information than by watching television. If a group of people is featured prominently on TV and is shown in a positive light, and the main characters in most shows come from that group, you can probably safely conclude that the group is valued by society and has power. Likewise, if you don't see a group, or they tend to be shown in peripheral or negative roles, you can conclude that this group lacks [influence] (2007, p. 150).

For example, *NCIS* offers two characters – Jethro Gibbs and Donald Mallard (affectionately referred to as Ducky) – who provide differing representations of ageing masculinity. Gibbs, the main character, exudes influence, whereas Ducky, a supporting character, is there largely to assist Gibbs. Team Leader Gibbs conforms to the ageing masculine hero motif – he is in charge, youthful, slim bodied and stylishly dressed – and thus represents 'successful' ageing (Hodgetts, Chamberlain, & Bassett, 2003, p. 419) and hegemonic masculinity. On the other hand, medical examiner Ducky corresponds to the motif of decline – his thinking appears muddled, his dress is dated, his body is sagging, and he is a carer (for his mother). Thus, Gibbs is highly competent and influential in the workforce, while Ducky is in some kind of time warp, continually going off on tangents, telling stories about his own youth and spouting irrelevant historical details. Despite this discrepancy, Ducky has a large fan following and is a frequent topic of discussion on the *Television Without Pity* forums.

Using the example of disability, Zola (1985) argues that analysis of minor characters is important analytical work that can offer insight into the social position of this group. We argue that the same can be said for characters who are old or fat, because both must navigate a disabling social world as well as (possible) body limitations. The tacit knowledge that surrounds disability, obesity and ageing provides a useful narrative prosthesis to programme makers and online audience discussions. Analysis of these internalized social statements offers an insight into the ways these groups have traditionally been symbolically annihilated and whether online audiences reinforce this tacit knowledge.

For example, Kathleen LeBesco (2006) uses Zola's framework to consider the representation of fat and disabled peripheral characters on the critically acclaimed HBO television series *The Sopranos*. For LeBesco, disability and the tacit knowledge that surrounds it have always featured in *The Sopranos* because the show begins with mob boss Tony Soprano visiting a psychologist to deal with an anxiety disorder. *The Sopranos* also makes use of a large number of minor characters with disability to provide information about major characters and storylines. These characters, from Beansie Gaeta, a pizzeria owner beaten to the point of paraplegia, to Tony's institutionalized Uncle Hercules, to Svetlana, an amputee Russian nurse caring for Tony's ailing mother, act as what Mitchell and Snyder (2000) describe as a 'narrative prosthesis'. They argue disability is central to narrative discourse and is used in a variety of ways:

> … as a character-making trope in the writer's arsenal, as a social category of deviance, as a symbolic vehicle for meaning-making and cultural critique, and as an option in the narrative negotiation of disabled subjectivity (p. 1).

In another example, the energetic online discussion about Sookie, a fat character on the *Gilmore Girls,* again highlights the importance of considering peripheral representations. The *Gilmore Girls* centres on single mother Loreli and her teenage daughter Rory. They talk fast, eat badly and drink too much coffee. Early episodes show Loreli and Rory eating fast food at Luke's Diner. Proprietor (and later fiancé to Loreli) Luke attempts to preach a healthy eating lifestyle to them by sneaking in light options and ignoring their orders for fatty food. Yet Loreli and Rory remain thin despite their unhealthy eating and lifestyles. In contrast to this, Loreli's best friend Sookie (Melissa McCarthy) is overweight. Sookie is a chef – she is knowledgeable and passionate about food. She is, however, a secondary character there only to support Loreli.

Gilmore Girls follows a tradition of representation that relies on secondary characters to add much of the atmosphere and narrative prosthesis regarding main characters. Although Sookie, as a secondary fat character, carries 'water for the svelte' Loreli (Lloyd, 2010), she breaks with tacit knowledge to a certain degree to offer an alternative representation of a fat woman. Indeed, without Sookie, perpetual failure Loreli would be unable to achieve her dream of running a restaurant.

Sookie has been hotly debated online for both her positive and negative qualities in relation to stereotypes of fat characters on television. The first image of Sookie in the series is of her falling over pots and pans and setting something on fire – a typical clumsy fat character focused on food. Contrarily, although she is criticized online for her peripheral status, she is (unlike Loreli) successful in her relationship and does champion a healthy eating message to offer an alternative representation of obesity on television:

> … there are also many positive things about her depiction. Sookie knows her food and cooks it herself. She has a joy of eating that is just as uninhibited as that of Lorelei and Rory, but it's mixed with a knowledge and appreciation of food that they don't have. For example, Sookie and her husband Jackson grow some of their own vegetables, while Lorelei never eats salad. These two attitudes on food can be seen as complimentary, because Sookie also enjoys unhealthy treats. She gets better nutrition, but there's no element of moral virtue in her eating. A fat woman who enjoys eating but is also mindful of nutrition and cooking is a positive rebuttal of stereotypes. Sookie isn't on a constant diet, and she isn't shown as either more gluttonous or more deprived than Lorelei (Deniselle, 2008).

The same is true in regards to the ageing body. Many older characters continue only to be represented in cameo roles on television. When these characters are in main roles, the programme is usually a documentary or lifestyle programme about old age such as *My Generation*, *Golden Oldies*, *When Teenage Meets Old Age* and *When I Get Older*. In *The Guardian* (Mangan, 2012) review of the documentary *When I Get Older*, the newspaper queried whether the BBC was serving older viewers properly. This idea of serving older viewers is interesting – documenting old age in shows like this continues to imply that audiences are young and that oldness is a kind of separate and pitiable or admirable/heroic state that television representations objectify. The programme makers' assumption that audiences are non-disabled, slim and young, with a high disposable income, is part of the normative formula that continues to dominate television representation and audience identification.

The online response to the *Guardian* article was mixed. However, very few posters cited particular entertainment programmes that featured older characters in main roles. The one exception was the programme *New Tricks*, as posted by TheChamp:

> New Tricks is a perfect example of something aimed at an older demographic which is a huge success. And for that reason the BBC hates it as it doesn't tick all those 18–35 boxes and is not beloved by the Mediaguardian and the rest of the chattering classes and therefore has no kudos …
>
> If only they realized the population is aging and it's those people who are staying in and watching the telly enjoying this stuff then they might be able to relax a bit (2012).

Apart from *New Tricks* – which centres on retired detectives re-employed by the force to solve cold cases – a couple of recent American legal dramas do have older people as main characters such as *Harry's Law* starring 64-year-old Kathy Bates, and *Boston Legal* starring 77-year-old William Shatner and 66-year-old Candice Bergen. Both programmes were created by David E. Kelly who is renowned for his atypical characters.

These representations and discussions draw on a long representational history of cultural omission, trivialization and condemnation. Although similarly pathologized and symbolically annihilated, each identity category – disability, obesity and ageing – has a different research history. Whereas disability researchers have concentrated on the ways disabled bodies are rejected as abnormal, critiques of fat characters on television focus on stereotypes, and ageing theorists analyse content largely on the basis of gender, as we outline below.

Representing Disability

For Paul Darke (2004, p. 100), the media's representation of disability has always been stereotypical, clichéd and archetypal, with representations focusing on impairment rather than society's disabling agenda. He argues normality is the key to understanding disability representation:

> Normality – the belief that there is essentially a correct way to have been born, look like and be – the belief in normality, has defined the nature of the

> representation of disability and impairment (and non-disability) by formulating it as the basis on which otherness […] has been defined in all figurative representation of humanity (pp. 103–104).

This belief in normality and use of disability as the basis for otherness is evident in cultural representations that precede the modern mass media. For example, along with the Bible (see passages such as Leviticus 21:16–20, Deuteronomy 27:27, John 5:14 and Matthew 9:2), there is a strong literary tradition that equates disability with punishment for evil – examples include *Frankenstein*, *Richard III*, Captain Hook and Captain Ahab. In addition to this conflation with evil, several clear stereotypes of disability emerge as a result of figurative representations, including people with disability as a source of humour, and people with disability as extraordinarily gifted (Gray, 2008, p. 111).

For both Gray (2008) and Luther, Ringer Lepre and Clark (2012), the most common images of disability on television see the character with disability being demeaned or laughed at. This stereotype can be traced through cultural representations that precede television. For example, Barnes observes that people with disability were often the source of ridicule in joke books of the Middle Ages (Barnes, 1997). This ridicule was extended during the 1600s when trips to Bedlam Hospital were a popular form of recreation amongst the wealthy who, according to Barnes (p. 15), also kept '"idiots" as objects of entertainment'. People with disability continued to be used as a source of humour, as human oddities, as court jesters and, notably, in freak shows (Haller, 2010).

The freak show, where biological rarities or so-called 'freaks of nature' performed in travelling circuses and carnivals for profit, is a canonical image of Western culture. They were a popular source of entertainment between 1840 and 1940 (Bogdan, 1990, p. 2). People with disability were also a key feature of the human curiosity shows which preceded the freak show as a form of entertainment during the 1700s. In this genre, bodies were constructed as spectacles and 'displayed in the context of popular entertainment' (Smith, 2005, p. 79). For Bogdan, people with disability were stylized and presented in a certain social context to *appear* as freaks – the discourse of the entertaining freak show thus constructed them as not normal and subjected these bodies to a particular gaze.

Filmic and televisual representations draw on this history of disability as human oddity and source of amusement through characters such as Ken in *A Fish Called Wanda*, the cartoon character Elmer Fudd, and frequent references to 'spastics' on *The Young Ones*. More recently, eccentric characters – for example Sheldon Cooper from *The Big Bang Theory* – approximate characteristics associated with disabilities such as autism as a narrative prosthesis to explore social mores (Patch, 2012).

A number of critical disability theorists (Barnes, 1992; Darke, 1998; Ellis, 2008; Longmore, 2003) have identified stereotypes and archetypes of disability often embraced by the media. Jack Nelson (2000, p. 184) summarizes these various stereotypical portrayals:

- the disabled person as victim: the focus of telethons
- the disabled person as hero: supercrip
- the disabled person as a threat: evil and threatening
- the disabled person as unable to adjust: 'just buck up'
- the disabled person as one to be cared for: the burden
- the disabled person as one who shouldn't have survived: better off dead.

Nelson argues that these images aid viewers in building an image of the world around them and contribute to what people think people with disability are really like. Disability is seen to exist in the realm of medicine which for Barnes also includes psychology, special education and social work (Barnes, 2004, p. 29). Under these so-called deficit models, disability is abnormal – a deviant or medical category – an undesirable tragedy that should be cured. These are clearly recognizable narratives that draw on a long tradition of representation, particularly in human interest stories. Narratives such as these tend to individualize disability as a personal problem (Ellis, 2009). Oliver (1990) argues that medical models see disability as an individual's problem caused by functional limitations or psychological losses.

Returning to the idea of Nelson's stereotypical list, it can be argued that, when it comes to the representation of disability, across programmes and genres, archetypal images emerge. The first archetypal image to emerge bestows characters with disability with superior knowledge by virtue of their disability (Gray, 2008, p. 111). As Rachael Leahcar, a contestant with vision impairment who competed in *The Voice* Australia (2012) and who is discussed further in the next chapter, comments, people with disability are viewed as extraordinary for doing ordinary things:

> My wish is for society to change their attitude towards disabilities. Some people say it's inspiring that someone with a disability can get on with their life as normal … but it would be nice if this was normal instead of inspiring. People seem to see the things that can't be done once you lose your sight, which there are many of. But what about the things you can do? Consider this, if there is a blackout, I'd be the only one in my house who could still manouvre around!! I use my other senses a lot more. I can hear/feel things that others cannot or don't notice because they rely on their sight more (2012).

This quote from Leahcar, although critiquing the archetype of the inspirational compensatory qualities of people with disabilities, arguably continues to perpetuate it.

Secondly, people with disability are a source of ridicule such as the plethora of strange characters adding an eerie atmosphere in the cult classic *Twin Peaks* (Space Crip, 2012). The enduring influence of this early 1990s cult drama can be seen in the way television dramas invoke strange peripheral characters to provide more information about the main characters. The narrative conceit that drove the two-season run of *Twin Peaks* was the murder of homecoming queen Laura Palmer. Both the town in which she is murdered and Dale Cooper – the FBI agent sent there to investigate – are more than they first appear. Blogger Space Crip (2012) describes the symbolic use of disability in *Twin Peaks* as a 'quirky town' narrative strategy, and identifies a number of characters that exhibit incidental, and oft-ridiculed, disabilities such as hearing impairment, blindness, wheelchair use, anxiety and Tourette syndrome. As Space Crip suggests, these intersect with both technical features and emotive influences:

> … difference (particularly difference in ability and race) is used to establish other-worldliness–a threatening other-worldliness that preys upon pretty white women (i.e., Laura Palmer, Maddy, Annie) and corrupts the souls and bodies of upstanding, middle-class white men (i.e., Philip Gerard, Leland Palmer, and Coop). Of course, Twin Peaks' handling of disability is not all bad. When looking at characters with disabilities on an individual basis, there are moments of transgression and rebellion against ableist stereotypes, but when looking at the disabled populations of Twin Peaks and Black Lodge as a whole, the mass of disabled bodies is used to create a mood of quirkiness and unease. Much like one would use lighting, sound, costuming, or set dressing.

Space Crip contends that 'quirky town' is now a well-established part of television's makeup, obvious in shows such as *Gilmore Girls*, *Lost*, *Carnivàle* and *Fringe*. Even shows which do not invoke this particular strategy make use of secondary characters, including some with disability, to provide insight into the main characters' motivations and world view. Disability continues to be a pervasive cultural image that serves a symbolic function across several formats and genres.

These televisual representations carry expectation and representational weight and are useful in understanding disability as a real concept and identity. Especially so when analysts ask what audiences do with them or what we consider the representations themselves are saying (Gray, 2008). When we recognize that bodies are interpreted through culture, disability can be thought of in a different way – as a socially dictated restriction imposed on certain bodies but not on others. This social restriction also applies to fat bodies, or those constructed as obese.

Representing the 'Fat' Body

Representing large body size or fat characters has a long history going back to the early political pamphleteers and advertisers for weight loss products (Farrell, 2011). One example is William Banting's 1863 pamphlet *Letter on Corpulence* which first appeared in England and, not long after, was reprinted in Europe and America (Huff, 2001, p. 39). Banting 'interpellates' (cited in Huff, p. 42) the reader as a fellow sufferer of obesity – that is, someone subjected to stares and stigma for not fitting the normal standard. It is assumed by Banting that the reader fears and wants to eradicate fat. Huff (pp. 42, 52) proposes that Banting's pamphlet is part of the common 'cultural discourse' that disparaged corpulent individuals for self-indulgent practices of excessive eating and drinking, as well as sedentary living.

In the nineteenth century, fat bodies were depicted in *Life* and *Harper's Weekly* magazines (Farrell, 2011, p. 29). For example, the portrayal of the 'fat cat' capitalist who was seen as a wealthy 'powerful man' because he (mostly male) had power over working people's lives (Farrell, pp. 29, 30; Mosher, 2001, p. 173). Modern day representations of the fat body in popular discourse on television have shifted emphasis, in that 'overweight' is now synonymous with 'unhealthy' (Heyes, 2007, p. 68); however, many of the old stereotypes still circulate in today's media. For instance, in a recent episode of *Mike & Molly*, 'Samuel gets Fired', the café owner Abe is depicted as a fat capitalist despite being smaller in size than both Mike and Molly.

In other cases, the 'fat cat' could be depicted as 'sinister, greedy and oppressive' (Farrell, 2011, pp. 29–32). Boss Hogg of *The Dukes of Hazzard* is a clear example of this. As a stereotypical corrupt public figure, Boss Hogg's weight acts as semiotic shorthand for his greed and laziness. Boss Hogg appeared in every episode of the long-running television show, always wearing a slightly-too-tight white suit, and always smoking a cigar as he engaged in criminal activities.

Another nineteenth-century approach was to depict fatness as a 'spectacle' – the corpulent fat person was displayed as a phenomenon in travelling shows, fairs and circuses (Farrell, 2011, pp. 32, 33). Indeed, fat bodies appeared alongside disabled bodies in freak shows in the context of popular entertainment. In early-twentieth century films, fat characters were typically in secondary roles or constructed as a foil for skinny characters who were also an oddity – a classic example of this is Laurel (the skinny one) being paired with Hardy who was 113 kg.

This stereotype of obesity being akin to a sideshow persists today. For example, the 2012 *The Biggest Loser: Singles* (Australia) participant Ryan who weighs-in at 241 kg is presented as the fattest man *ever* on the programme, *in the world.* Using an incredulous tone, the personal trainers speak of Ryan as a specimen, to use Farrell's words, of 'human grotesquery' (2011, p. 32). Another recent example is the programme *My Big Fat Fetish* which presents big beautiful women Reenaye, Kitt, Lizzie and Patty and their consumption of food as a spectacle. The four women are super-sized models with weight ranging between 114–280 kg. The participants on the programme gain weight to pose for videos, magazines and online websites. They eat foods high in carbohydrates, sugars and fats (most often found in fried foods) because it is the fastest way to gain weight. Eating food on *My Big Fat Fetish* also becomes spectacle, and although the programme claims to examine the lifestyle of the four super-sized models, they remain spectacles. Their bodies are marvelled at, they are treated as novelties and stylized by the camera's gaze to invoke feelings of disgust. Like Ryan in *The Biggest Loser*, Patty (at 280 kg) is a manipulated televisual specimen of human grotesquery.

Some studies claim that the more prevalent stereotypes of fat bodies position fat characters as the butt of slim characters' jokes and as a way to ridicule certain social categories and to signify inferiority (Farrell, 2011, p. 32; Murray, 2007, p. 363). Billy Bunter (Richards, 1908), the corpulent early-twentieth century public school boy weighing about 90 kg, exemplifies this stereotype. Although not considered heavy by *The Biggest Loser* standards, Bunter's weight was substantial at a time when most people in England did not have enough to eat. Bunter frequently talks about food – namely treacle, oranges, cake – he has pilfered from others or has hoarded himself. On the BBC programme *Billy Bunter of Greyfriars School*, Bunter was played for comedic effect and often mocked by the other peripheral characters.

Cartoons in popular culture such as those in *Life* magazine also used large-sized bodies as a signifier of inferiority to caricature middle class changes in social levels during the early 1900s (Farrell, 2011). Farrell (p. 41) contends that such cartoons, 'mocked middle-class white fat people for too excessively indulging in the pleasures and freedoms that had been ushered in during the advent of the modern era'. These depictions were signifiers of middle-class fat men and women as lacking self-discipline and self-control in their attempts to improve themselves and their lifestyle (Farrell, pp. 41–42). Middle class men were doubly derided for attempting upward mobility such as furthering their education; examples include images of fat men with captions such as 'Self-Taut' (p. 43). They were also depicted, like Boss Hogg, bulging out of ill-fitting dress suits, which signified 'how ill-suited they were for the pleasures of the rich' (p. 43).

The same was true for women. Middle-class women's increased wealth enabled them to travel and pursue leisure activities but, because they overindulged in eating and drinking, many became portly (Farrell, 2011, p. 52). The stout women were seen to lack the discipline needed to control their weight – that is, they lacked the class of aristocratic women who maintained a svelte body into middle and older age. Invoked here is the idea that the civilized body is thin, an idea that persists in twenty-first century television media. This middle-class idea was evident when celebrity chef Jamie Oliver in his programme *Jamie's Ministry of Food* described Rotherham mother Julie Critchlow as a 'fat scrubber' for passing hamburgers through the school gates to her children rather than encouraging them to participate in Oliver's healthy eating campaign.

Fat bodies have been associated with a number of negative qualities such as laziness, badness, dirtiness, ugliness, greediness, social unattractiveness and gluttony – these values are tacit knowledge repurposed from earlier media. Recent television representations take this tacit knowledge further to portray fat characters as being passive, sexually inept, rarely in a romantic relationship, having poor personal hygiene, and engaging in clichéd eating patterns. For instance, the peripheral character Norm in *Cheers* fits the image of the passive, lazy, unattractive and sexually inept character. Norm sits at the bar complaining about life, politics, losing his job and how dissatisfied he is with his wife Vera. Norm is played for comedic effect through his large body size and one liner comments such as joining a gym because it has an 'excellent snack bar'.

Representing Ageing

Traditionally, older characters on television have been in the minority; however, this has been for different reasons than for disabled and obese characters. Signorielli (2001) concluded that 89 per cent of people represented on television are in the age range of 18–50 years. People in this age range are considered to have 'more disposable income' by television producers and advertisers – in short, this age group has more money to spend and thus television is populated with representations of this group (p. 35). Perhaps not surprisingly, older men appear on television more often than older women (about six men to four women), yet 51 per cent of the population in the US are women (Bradley & Longino, 2001, p. 19; Signorielli, 2001). Studies do not explain why there is a gender bias; however, the most obvious reason is that older male characters are depicted in powerful roles. Most of the older women who appear on television are portrayed as younger than their actual characters' age (Signorielli, 2004, p. 296).

Long before the advent of television, ageing bodies were caricatured by cartoonists in several ways: 'deep lines on the face and loose skin beneath the chin' and 'shorter distance between nose and chin (if false teeth have been removed)'; a 'loss of hair or gray hair'; and 'liver spots on the hands, bowed legs, and stooped backs' (Scarfe cited in Bradley & Longino, 2001, p. 18). Cartoonists also used signifiers of old age such as glasses, 'walking canes, walkers, or wheelchairs' (p. 18) to ridicule the elderly. In the televisual world of today, not much has altered. Physical signs of ageing such as 'grey hair', 'wrinkles and ailments' are consistently used by programme makers as visual 'shorthand' to connote a decaying, declining body close to death (Chivers, 2011, p. xix). Televisual images of this kind are being used to a lesser degree but they are still used to evoke a set response.

Like depictions of disability and obesity, stereotyping ageing relies on tacit knowledge to create socially disabling attitudes about what it means to be old. Prior to the early 1980s only a few programmes featured older people as the main characters. Those older people who did appear were either depicted in demeaning ways or their bodies were portrayed as declining and decaying (Vernon, Williams, Phillips, & Wilson, 1991). For example, they were more likely than other characters in the programme to be represented as 'comical, stubborn, eccentric, and foolish' (Bell, 1992, p. 306). Furthermore, older characters were shown as being 'treated with disrespect' as well as deprived and suffering (Davis & Davis cited in Bell, 1992, p. 306). For these and other reasons, Signorielli (2004, p. 299) concludes that 'being old on television is not a very enviable position, particularly for women and minorities'.

As might be expected, there is a discrepancy between the way older male and female characters are represented on television. Typically, male characters between the ages of 50–64 are predominantly white and in high status positions such as a doctor, lawyer, business man, or chief detective (Bradley & Longino, 2001, p. 19; Signorielli, 2001, p. 36; Signorielli, 2004, p. 297). However, male characters over 65 years are often typecast in 'jobs that are not particularly prestigious' (Signorielli, 2004, p. 297). Women over the age of 50, however, are rarely depicted as working outside the home; Signorielli (2001, p. 36) found only 12.7 per cent were portrayed as working in professions. Thus, female characters were seen to be on the periphery, despite the attention television has historically given to extended family life in dramas, soap operas and situation comedies.

For example, in *Dallas* (1978–1991), a long-running and top-rating primetime drama, male actors are the protagonists, even though the relationships between the Ewing family members play a major part in the series. Over the series it is J.R. Ewings' exploits as a greedy oil baron, his dysfunctional marriage and his business differences with his brother Bobby that drive the plot. The male characters portray business men as harbingers of power. The older woman in the series, J.R.'s mother, is the archetypical ageing matriarch. Throughout the series, the other female characters – Sue Ellen Ewing, Miss Ellie Ewing, Pamela Barnes Ewing – are located within the domestic and social spheres in support of the main male characters.

The idea that women must 'remain youthful', while men are likely to 'show signs of aging', is perpetuated by television casting (Vernon et al., 1991, p. 66). This tendency is evident in many peripheral characters such as Molly's mother Joyce in *Mike & Molly* played by 68-year-old actress Swoosie Kurtz, and Charlie's mother Evelyn in *Two and a Half Men* played by 69-year-old actress Holland Taylor.

These youthful–older women are slim bodied, stylishly dressed and sexually available. Arguably this stereotype emanated from television characters such as Blanche Devereaux (played by 51-year-old Rue McClanahan) from *The Golden Girls* and Samantha Jones (played by 42-year-old Kim Cattrall) from *Sex and the City*.

However, the general televisual characterization of ageing has changed since the 1980s. Older people have been represented in more diverse ways, in particular as more active, as socially engaged, as mentally astute, as physically healthy and as pursuing meaningful work. Bell (1992, pp. 307–309), in his study of five primetime television programmes of the late 1980s and early 1990s – *Matlock*, *The Golden Girls*, *Jake and the Fatman*, *Murder, She Wrote* and *In the Heat of the Night* – revealed that each featured characters over 60 years of age who were central rather than peripheral to the action, were functioning in powerful and influential roles and were admired by other characters. Interestingly, all the older characters either had professional jobs such as detectives or crime fiction writers, or had independent means. However, Bell noted that characters and storylines were still attached to a mythic 'old order' – that is, linked to patriarchal and individualistic values (pp. 308–310).

Bell concluded that primetime television does not know how to represent ongoing intimate relationships between older men and older women. Older characters, in the 60-year-old age range are generally not depicted as engaging in sexual activity on television. So, while older characters may be attractive, flirtatious or sexy – a common thread across the programmes Bell studied – they are not portrayed in sexual scenes (1992, p. 309). Specifically, older characters are not shown as touching in erotic ways and as being sexually 'satisfied' (1992, p. 309). For instance, the programme *As Time Goes By* portrays two older characters who are involved in a romantic relationship. However, they have a lack of sexual activity, as signified by their pyjama wearing in bed – sexual activity for this couple happened when they were lovers at the time of the Korean War.

In addition, in programmes such as *One Foot in the Grave*, older people are often portrayed as grumpy. Yet, with a twist, grumpiness is celebrated in the *Grumpy Old Men* and *Grumpy Old Women* series, and on affiliated websites such as Seniors.gov.au and ABC message board. Postings to these online forums recognize and appreciate the reworking of the tired grumpy archetype, as illustrated by the following sample:

> I enjoy it. It's like having my grumpy old friends around for a cuppa and a critique of … just about everything, actually! (Austral ®, 2010).

> I liked 'Grumpy Old Men' as well, but I must say that I really like 'Grumpy Old Women'. I think they are so clever and straight about how they feel. I enjoy watching them very much (beetle, 2005).

However, programme makers reclaiming a stereotype can rebound on the particular social group because some audiences endorse the archetype – in this case of the grumpy old person – by continuing to laugh and poke fun at older people. We therefore argue that the value of this online discussion is not limited to celebrating or reclaiming a stereotype, but extends to its '*use*' (Gray, 2008, p. 114). The *Grumpy Old* series could be recognized as starting a conversation about the process of growing older – a conversation that has overflowed onto the online forums. Many online audiences' responses to the series correspond with our point of view. Even though that conversation is more celebratory than critical, some online participants identified with, but, at the same time, disliked the representations:

> More than the personalities themselves, what ired me was the negative presentation. If I truly desired to hear such acrimonious rubbish I'd make a tape of myself (earle qaeda ®, 2010b).

We argue that it's not a matter of whether grumpy is a positive or a negative image of old age, nor if it is about reclaiming a stereotype – rather we are concerned with how the image is mobilized in the context of online forums where participants negotiate identifications about older age. The following section discusses online audience activity as both evidence of active audiences and a progression of cultural representation.

Representational Weight: Viewing and Discussing

As Gray (2008, p. 115) notes of television entertainment, 'the weight of representation lies not only in any given television programme, but also in the use and discussion of that program'. The action of interrogating the representational system of television and its accompanying websites can produce significant public ideological intervention. However, we are cautious not to divide the representation into a positive and negative binary opposition. According to Snyder and Mitchell representations are inevitably 'bound to their own historical moment's shortcomings, idiosyncrasies, and obsessions' (2006, p. 201). Thus, what is considered positive now may not be so in the future. Therefore, although online discussions do veer towards describing some representations as positive and others negative, throughout this book we focus on whether audiences demonstrate, through the web, that they identify with the characters, situations and storylines offered on television as part of their negotiation with tacit knowledge.

From our analysis of online audiences engaging with television images of disability, obesity and ageing, we conclude that selected forums accessed by members of the public have the potential to provide 'public deliberation' (Mummery & Rodan, 2011, p. 300). Regular viewers – those likely to watch each episode of a programme and who may go beyond watching the programme to participate in online discussions – have been examined in several academic studies (Andrejevic, 2008; Brooker, 2004; Costello & Moore, 2007; Jones, 2003; Ross, 2009); however, regular viewers who go online to participate in discussions about disability, obesity and ageing on television have not been interrogated to the same degree. One exception is Quinlan and Bates's (2008) content analysis of journalistic and blogger reactions to Heather Mills's performance (a contestant with a disability) on *Dancing with the Stars* (USA). Quinlan and Bates (2008) argue that an exploration of the user-generated critical response demonstrates the ways disability operates within culturally based paradigms. Audience response to representations of ageing and obesity are subject to similar culturally based paradigms.

The availability of online responses to television representations of disability, obesity and ageing furnish academic researchers with a rich database for their analysis of these groups and the ways they figure on television and, by extension, in public discourse. Bronwyn Williams (2009) observes that participatory online spaces allow viewers and online forum members from disparate audience demographics to come together and assist each other in making meaning from texts. According to Williams (pp. 38, 42), in these online shared spaces individuals can potentially connect instantaneously to others who have similar interests. Interests flourish and impressions can develop from engaging with others' ideas and the inevitable tensions that emerge in most online discussions. Viewers can test half-formed ideas, ask questions and evaluate forum members' replies. Indeed, a great deal of the content posted on official generated and unofficial generated sites about televisual texts pivots 'on interpretive questions' (p. 39). These conversations which are in effect interpreting representations become a form of representation themselves. A representation that conveys social attitudes regarding disability, obesity and ageing.

Conclusion

Viewers draw on tacit knowledge – internalized social statements they hear in the televisual media and in everyday life – about disabled, old and obese people. This tacit knowledge is a pervasive narrative prosthesis across several formats and genres. Online audiences draw on representations within programmes and talk about these with co-workers, family, friends and online; they also read about these in magazines, newspapers and in social media. Online discussions are intertextual texts which draw on each other as well as cultural histories of representation to produce particular versions of reality (cf. Couldry, 2000).

As we have demonstrated throughout this chapter, cultural representations of disability, obesity and ageing have historically presented these groups as lacking social power – they are rejected bodies subject to disabling stereotypes and archetypes. They have been subject to a symbolic annihilation through representations which omit, trivialize and condemn the existence of these groups. For example, people with disability have been a source of ridicule; obesity has carried with it cultural associations with gluttony, immorality and spectacle; ageing has been considered in terms of dependence and decline. Yet all of these groups are encouraged to exhibit an ideal positive personal attitude and ignore their socially constructed pathologization.

The next chapter continues the discussion of the importance of online discourse as a cultural text. We consider several themes which online audiences focus on when discussing the televisual representation of disability, obesity and ageing, including stereotypes and misrepresentation, quantification, 'that's not something I want to see!', and, finally, 'I like this'. We argue that these online spaces are both reflective of and resistant towards the social disablement experienced by people who are disabled, old and obese.

Chapter 3

A Marketplace of Ideas: Television as a Social Experience

> [Television] focuses our most prevalent concerns, our deepest dilemmas. Our most traditional views, those that are repressive and reactionary, as well as those that are subversive and empancipatory, are upheld, examined, maintained, and transformed (Newcombe & Hirsch, 1994, p. 506).

> As someone who was a chubby kid, a fat teen and now a chubby twenty-something, I am always wary of the two brands of fat portrayal on television: the wise-crackin' crying shoulder (Sookie on *Gilmore Girls*) and the tragic cautionary whale (Carmen on *Popular*). The part I dislike the most, though, is that there never seemed to be any happy medium between skinny and huge: chubby is almost never an area that TV knows what to do with, needing instead to rush to extremes to make their point (Arboleda, 2010).

Television is a technology, a piece of furniture and a means of mass communication. As Newcombe and Hirsch note in the quote at the head of the chapter, television offers the opportunity for dissent while also possessing the power to maintain the status quo. Televisual images constitute 'a "marketplace of ideas" where political issues can be publicly debated' (Lorié, 2011, p. 36). Although these images may reflect society's desire for change they are also ideologically encoded and offer messages about identity and social value. Sarah Arboleda's critique above of television's binary approaches to fat characters is typical of the way the discussion and debate that Lorié refers to increasingly takes place on online forums, blogs and websites. Indeed, many people mobilize online to voice their opinion about various television representations. This outpouring of audience writing and appraising of images, dialogue and technical production is unprecedented in the history of television.

This chapter focuses on the ways televisual representations of disability, obesity and ageing are being publicly debated online. We consider activist sites initiated by a number of social justice movements affiliated with disability, seniors, fat acceptance and feminism and those – both official and unofficial – that emerge from particular television programmes. These web forums are important sites for viewers to struggle with televisual images that integrate body ideals with our idea of what is physically 'normal' (Wendell, 1996, p. 91).

This is particularly relevant to bodies deemed disabled, obese and old because each has been rejected as socially unacceptable or abnormal through television representations.

We begin the chapter with a discussion of the emergence of online conversations about television texts, with a particular focus on what Sharon Ross (2009, p. 4) has termed 'tele-participation'. According to Ross, tele-participation is the invitation by television networks for viewers to interact with programmes 'beyond the moment of viewing and "outside" of the show itself' by participating in online activity (p. 4). We consider the ways images of disability, obesity and ageing are publicly discussed and debated on online forums. This section divides the discussion between official forums, activist websites/blogs, and finally unofficial forums that do not have any particular allegiance to activist groups. The second section of the chapter explores the common themes that emerge in online discussion of televisual representations of disability, obesity and ageing to examine how dominant discourses of disability, obesity and ageing are being contested and/or reinforced and whether this aligns with academic critiques of these representations. We divide the discussion into four thematic trends – stereotypes and misrepresentation, quantification, 'that's not something I want to see!', and, finally, 'I like this'. We argue that through these discussions, online audiences ask interpretive questions to introduce critiques and new ways of thinking about disability, obesity and ageing. The final part of the chapter considers the symbolic power operating within the television show *The Voice* Australia (2012) and the surrounding social media discourse as online audiences publicly debate political issues regarding representations of disability, obesity and ageing. *The Voice* initiates a tele-participation which in turn reveals insights into the ways ordinary viewers both contest and reinforce dominant discourses of disability, obesity and ageing.

The Invitation to Interact Online

For television networks now, any television website that viewers interact with – whether official or viewer-generated – supports the television networks' strategy to keep viewers 'engaged after the program ends' (Gillan, 2011, p. 59). Gillan argues that 'flow is more circular with each platform' – whether it is the television programme, the website or the mobile device, network television convinces viewers to get into one more platform with the hope that they 'return to the on-air text' (p. 76). Official sites attempt to engage audiences and in doing that 'increase loyalty to a show or brand' as well as simultaneously cross-promote other programmes (Deery, 2003, pp. 163–164). Similarly, although unofficial sites may have no authorized relationship with the on air programme, they still offer exposure and further brand engagement.

Building on Hall's model of encoding and decoding, viewers rarely actively withdraw from the media, nor are they so accepting of the images presented. In fact, audiences are often openly sceptical about media representations. Viewers engage with televisual media on multiple levels and exhibit a variety of responses, from irony to scepticism to a willingness to suspend disbelief (Couldry, 2000, p. 9). Online audiences doubt many claims made on television and alert other viewers to framing techniques used by programme makers. Indeed viewers are often self-reflexive about their own use of programmes. Yet even when online audiences are aware of the way television shapes particular concepts of disability, obesity and ageing, they may draw on disabling tacit knowledge to adopt and perpetuate these views.

The online audience is offered the illusion that they are having a 'meaningful interaction' on official websites, thereby adding to the viewing event (Jones, 2003, p. 401). For some online audiences, being aware that one is watching a programme 'with identifiable others', with whom the programme can be discussed in detail during and/or after the airing, creates anticipation while watching. During this exchange of views online, a viewer's outlook could be transformed (Williams, 2009).

This possibility for transformation affects the viewing experience. We argue that this happens in different ways, depending on the forum in which the interaction takes place. Although we discuss online audiences in the broadest sense throughout this book, it is important to make a distinction between viewer-generated content and official-generated content television websites. A further distinction must be made between viewer-generated sites and social activist sites, which are also viewer-generated, but have clear and specific goals about transforming the media or improving the social position of a particular group such as the disabled, old or obese. As discussed in the previous chapter, whereas disability, obesity and ageing have traditionally been negated forms of subjectivity, rejected as undesirable bodies, they are now popular televisual fascinations. Yet their image continues to be informed by disabling tacit knowledge derived from earlier cultural representations. As the Internet and World Wide Web secures its place in our televisual and media experience, the way these identifications are publicly debated online in both official and unofficial forms offers an insight into the ways this tacit knowledge persists through emerging forms of cultural representation despite a supposedly more enlightened social environment. The next section considers the materialization of online participation or tele-participation as an integral part of the televisual experience.

Tele-participation and Official v Unofficial Sites

Viewer official or unofficial websites have three functions: one function is to enable viewers to chat about a programme in 'a many-to-many mode'; the second is to provide information about the programme such as characters, episodes, writers, directors etc.; and the third is to allow viewers and visitors to purchase merchandise allied with the programme (Deery, 2003, p. 164). Whereas early research on television viewing with programme websites focused on fan cultures and on the extent to which viewers participated in the websites beyond the television programme (Jenkins, 1992), this book does not concern itself specifically with fan cultures. We do, however, agree with Jenkins (pp. 277–278) that online audiences exhibit both 'emotional proximity and critical distance'. Tele-participation is emerging as an important feature of the television viewing experience for particular audience demographics. For example, reviewers of popular television shows now draw on online discussions as a way to gauge public reaction. We similarly use this representation of public reaction and opinion throughout this book to gauge social attitudes regarding disability, obesity and ageing.

Online audiences engage and interact with official-generated and viewer-generated websites. Most official television websites, as well as many viewer-generated ones, are open public forums, which can be accessed by both viewers and non-viewers. We refer to official websites as those that are affiliated with the television production in question. They form part of the production itself with the on air text explicitly encouraging audiences to further engage with content online. These sites may include discussion forums, character biographies, episode descriptions, a media section outlining news about the cast, crew and show, and a shop from which to purchase official merchandising.

Most viewers access official websites to find out information and purchase merchandise (Brooker, 2004, p. 578) – thus the focus is mainly on consumerism both for the viewer and the television station. Early television companion websites focused on 'building audience relationships' for the programme (Ross, 2009, p. 9) by inviting audiences onto websites to participate in competitions, commentary and voting. These relationships, as a form of circular flow, were designed to yield advertising dollars (Deery, 2003, p. 162).

Prior to the formation of the read–write web in 2004, most discussion took place on official forums which predominately operated as information resources or merchandising outlets. However, with web 2.0, an environment emerged whereby people became more likely to go beyond contributing to programme websites by creating their own. This technological advancement has made a huge difference to the amount and level of discussions taking place on official-generated and viewer-generated websites. Discussions on these sites tend to be interactive and various as threads/topics emerge; furthermore, these discussions are not limited to people's favourite characters. Web 2.0 has also precipitated the rise of social activist groups with large online followings.

Other unofficial sites are created and frequented by those who watch the programme. Unofficial sites may take the form of dedicated audience response discussion boards such as *Television Without Pity* and *Whirlpool*, they may be an individual's blog site or they may form part of a larger social justice movement such as the fat acceptance *Big Fat Blog* or disability social justice *Feminists With Disability for a Way Forward* (FWD). Unofficial forums act as spaces for online audiences to engage with television texts outside of the moderation confines imposed on official forums.

Unofficial forums are particularly important to disability, obesity and ageing because they provide an alternative point of view. Similarly they may introduce critiques that have traditionally been relegated to the periphery of mainstream media attention. Nevertheless, official forums remain popular sites for tele-participation and discussion about televisual representations of disability, obesity and ageing.

Official Sites

According to Deery (2003, p. 165), official television programme websites are 'more closed and fixed' – the structure of the website is standard, open for the duration of the programme, participants cannot upload video nor hyperlinks, and discussion is moderated. In Brooker's study of *Dawson's Creek* he found that official sites tended to be reused as 'an information resource', because they are 'seen as more professional and reliable' (2004, p. 577). However, often the official website is archived at the end of the season, so viewers can no longer access it on the Internet. This limits discussion to the period during which the television broadcast takes place. Television producers are also able to limit the discussion according to their own agendas on official sites.

Moderation is a key feature of official television sites. Acting as a logical companion to the television programme itself, discussion threads are likely to reinforce the discourse offered within the programme. Although aspects of the programme may be criticized, including, for example, the behaviour of participants or characters, it is clear that these characters are constructed in particular ways to initiate audience involvement and therefore exposure to merchandising. As we discuss in the next chapter, characters constructed on-screen as disidentification targets continue to operate within the circular flow of enticing audiences to return to the on air text. Gray (2008) describes these sites as 'overflow' and an important part of the viewing experience. For Gray, viewers' engagement with television is no longer confined to television itself because viewers are invited to immerse themselves in the show online (p. 73).

Increasingly too, television producers rely on social media applications like Facebook and Twitter to maintain the circular flow of viewers. These platforms may be favoured by audience members because they are already using them and they allow discussion after the programme ends. For example, New Zealand viewers of *The Voice* Australia (discussed at the end of the chapter) were able to continue discussing official videos on YouTube even though *The Voice* was no longer airing in Australia.

Unofficial Sites

Although still a form of television overflow, unofficial sites can be distinguished from official sites as they do not have any particular affiliation with the on air text. Instead, these viewer-generated sites are created by people who have some attachment with the programme topic. Visitors either join a community on the topic, or they are activists who want to critique it. Deery found that viewer-generated websites 'tend to be open' and 'evolving' (2003, p. 165) – these sites allow the uploading of articles, videos and hyperlinks, and discussion can take off in different directions. Because these sites are not moderated to the same extent as official forums, unofficial forums adopt a less constrained tone. For example, discussants of *The Biggest Loser: Singles* (2012) contestant with a disability – Selena – on the official *Biggest Loser* forum, although expressing disappointment with the character, maintained a certain degree of respect. By comparison, discussants on the unofficial site *Whirlpool* were often cruel. Selena, was often depicted as unmotivated and struggling on *The Biggest Loser*. As a result, a large number of the online audience members also interpreted her as unmotivated. For instance, WORMGERM (2012) described Selena as a 'useless sack of crap'; vastmuse (2012) said, 'You dont wanna see what she has been shovelling in her pie hole since she has left, but i can assure you its probably carb loaded and saturated in fat'; and Judochop87 (2012) added, 'Selena is such a dumb bitch, she's so flapped in the head!' Such comments would be removed if posted on official sites that tend to have clear moderation policies. For example, discussants of the official *Biggest Loser* discussion forum must adhere to the following moderation policy:

> Like any social situation, there are simple rules and protcols that you should follow. Don't abuse people (your membership will be cancelled). Don't swear. Don't give out personal information (for your own security). And most of all, don't discuss anything that is illegal. It's mostly common sense, but there are always bad apples. If you see them, make sure you report them by clicking 'report abuse', that way they can be warned or banned, and the post can be removed ('Frequently Asked Questions', n.d.)

We analyse the ways Selena is constructed as an identification target in the following chapter.

Activist Sites

Social activist groups affiliated with the rejected identities discussed throughout this book have turned online to collaborate, discuss and critique televisual representation. Their tele-participation goes beyond television overflow and strives to change people's attitudes and the media itself. Online activist sites associated with fat acceptance and disability that engage with television and popular culture are popular online destinations. The fat acceptance movement, for example, is motivated to fight back against discrimination and what they see as the misrepresentation of obesity within government policies and legislation, the media, and diet industries' support of medical studies as well as their promotion of diet products.

Similarly, disability activism is characterized by an unwillingness to perform comfortable ableist stereotypes of individual suffering (Siebers, 2002, p. 41). The FWD popular culture blog is motivated to 'promot[e] discussion, conversation, fellowship, and education' ('About', n.d.). FWD articles frequently engage with television representations on a deep level to reveal the ways disability is culturally constructed to perpetuate a disabling prejudice.

Although these activists make important critiques about the ways obesity and disability are frequently represented on television, it is unclear what these bloggers would approve of because acceptable representations are rarely recognized. By comparison, discussants on senior social movement sites often engage in an appreciation of particular discourses of ageing on television. For instance, the American Association of Retired Persons (AARP) online members' forums devoted to television programmes have three groups – 'My Favorite TV Shows', 'Great PBS Programming' and 'Betty White fan Club'. AARP is a non-profit, non-partisan organization that assists people 50 years and older to 'have independence, choice and control in ways that are beneficial and affordable to them and society as a whole' ('About us', n.d.). AARP does not describe itself as an activist group in the same way as the disability and fat acceptance movements, although, interestingly, AARP now also funds and produces its own television programme, *My Generation* – a magazine, lifestyle programme targeted at 50 plus viewers, which covers health, money, relationship and volunteering issues. AARP might be best described as a lobby group for seniors.

Media activist websites are communicative spaces where groups can gather and offer alternative representations (Rodan & Balnaves, 2010). However, the impact of a community accessing the media is not the same as the mainstream media – often communities who censure the media for perpetuating stereotypes are also likely to be criticized in the mainstream press and by bloggers who perpetuate the major tropes and negative stereotypes of disability, obesity and ageing. For instance, when accessibility was explored in the Season 1 *Glee* episode 'Wheels' the response from disability bloggers was in radical opposition to the mainstream media. Whereas disability bloggers responded negatively to the depiction of disability as exploitative and tokenistic (see s.e. smith, 2009), the mainstream media interpreted the investigation of disability access issues as sensitive and empowering. Some even criticized the opinions of the disability activists (see Kennedy, 2009; Sheppard, 2011).

Television and Participatory Websites

Our discussion of online audience engagement with televisual images of disability, obesity and ageing throughout this book reveals several thematic trends. These trends – a concern with stereotypes and perceived misrepresentation, quantification, and whether or not the images are enjoyable to watch – reflect a desire for social change regarding disability, obesity and ageing but also reinforce ideologically encoded messages about the subjugation of these groups. As such, we argue these themes are political and illustrate a negotiation of televisual content.

The thematic trends, discussed in depth below, are also reflected in academic literature about the televisual representation of these groups. For example, Barnes (1992) lists several stereotypes of disability; Longmore (1987) calls for more realistic portrayals of disability; Richardson (2010) suggests disability is context specific; and Hevey (1997) recognizes the potential for audiences to recoil in disgust from representations of disability and the manner in which this response can be leveraged for social change.

Likewise, Murray (2005b, p. 155), identifies stereotypes of fat people and suggests audiences tend to read representations of fat bodies as disgusting. Richardson (2010) claims that what is considered fat in one context may not be in another. Gingras (2005, p. 255) calls for 'size acceptance' as a way of presenting more realistic images of older people; whereas, Ross and Moorti (2005, p. 84) call for 'alternative messages, narratives and images' to counteract the slim is ideal media message.

Similarly, Featherstone and Wernick (1995) list stereotypes of older people, and Bell (1992, p. 311) calls for older characters to appear more often and in 'more diverse' roles. Likewise, Healey and Ross (2002) recognize the need for more diverse images and representations of older people in television programming. Both yearn for more realistic portrayals of older people. Donlon et al. (2005, p. 315) argue for increasing older people's awareness of the 'unrealistic' depictions of the old on television. Hepworth (2000) maintains that if analysts scrutinize programming for its ability (or not) to present ageing as a process of change, their work would challenge existing stereotypes.

Thus the themes considered important to discuss by online audiences are also reflected in academic investigations of televisual representations of disability, obesity and ageing. Although some of the themes we identify, such as investigating stereotypes and realism, are increasingly criticized as modes of analysis in the academic literature, online audiences continue to find them useful. Whereas these themes emerge in most online discussion forums at some point or another, critiques of stereotypes and misrepresentation most frequently take place on activist sites and celebrations of characters or storylines appear on official and unofficial forums. These discussions reveal much about whether audiences identify with characters and by extension, the ways audiences contest or accept the vision of the world being offered by the television show.

Stereotypes and Misrepresentation

Online audiences are particularly aware of the construction of stereotypes. As we discussed in the previous chapter, disability, obesity and ageing carry a legacy of adverse cultural associations, and as a consequence audiences often disidentify with these topics and representations. Just as blogger Sarah Arboleda (2010) comments in the quote at the head of this chapter, theorists such as Richardson (2010) find that representations of fat characters on television tend to ascribe to stereotypes. Similarly, the observation that people with disability are constructed as either inspirational or tragic (Ellis & Goggin, 2014) is often noted by disability bloggers critically assessing the media (Haller, 2010). Indeed, people critiquing the representation of older people online also observe stereotypes that have been identified by academic theorists. For example, older characters are often portrayed as senile and sexless (Featherstone & Wernick, 1995).

This drive to critique stereotypes and misrepresentation can be seen in the reaction to *Britain's Missing Top Model*, a reality television show which claims to 'challeng[e] our ideas of beauty'. However, the focus on normalcy and beauty within this modelling competition for contestants with disability, alienated sections of the audience, as Jacki Brown articulates on the disability forum *Ramp Up*:

> … most of what I saw was the perpetuation of disability stereotypes, particularity the disability-as-personal-tragedy refrain, and contestants who were trying to squeeze into the narrow, and overdone cultural construct of female beauty … We already exist outside the dominate culture. Shouldn't we use that to express versions of sexuality that are exciting and haven't been overdone, that truly challenge ideas and are interesting for 'us' to watch as well? Britain's Missing Top Model is just pandering to white, straight, able-boded notions of what is acceptable (2011).

Similarly, participants on the *Big Fat Blog* identify several stereotypes about obesity that circulate in the media such as the view that people who are obese lack self-control and cannot resist food. Bloggers on this site often complain of damaging stereotypes about fat and obesity presented in *The Biggest Loser*.

Whereas *The Biggest Loser* is often critiqued for perpetuating stereotypical views of people who are obese as being unable to resist food, the situation comedy *Mike & Molly* purports to offer a more empowering representation by having two fat characters in the lead roles. However, even in *Mike & Molly* the main characters, Mike and Molly, frequently make references to high sugar foods such as cake, donuts, jam, cream and chocolate sundaes. In addition, the couple met at Overeaters Anonymous and as a consequence talking about food is central to each episode. As such Bilt4Cmfrt is sceptical about *Mike & Molly* on the *Big Fat Blog*:

> I'm looking at you 'Mike and Molly' which is starting to smell like, yet more sitcom droppings … Prove me wrong guys and I'll endorse you from the rooftops but I'm not holding my fat breath (2010).

Critiques about stereotypes frequently refer to how 'unrealistic' the representation is, or how it does not confer with the poster's own life experience. For example, online viewers of *Vera*, the police detective series, take this view on *The Guardian* television review site. *Vera*, played by Brenda Blethyn, is a middle-aged DCI – her character Vera Stanhope is a solitary and meticulous investigator who uses her experience, intuition, and knowledge of the Northumbria district to solve crimes. Some online viewers herald this detective show as offering a realistic 'middle-aged' female character:

> Brenda … is amazing. And how refreshing to see a rounded, middle-aged female character on TV (autostradas, 2011).

Similarly, Zoe Williams in her review for *The Guardian* (2011) describes Vera Stanhope as a believable middle-aged character, due to her remarkable 'sharpness' in her 'wits', and her 'desire to concentrate'. Yet, online audiences equally found the character Vera – and the casting of Brenda Blethyn – 'unrealistic' and 'unbelievable' (mugclass, 2011). For instance, Jackie (2011) said Vera came across as 'more like a neurotic granny than a police inspector'; klouise (2011) described the character as 'nothing more than a bumbling fool masquerading as a detective', who 'appeared half-cut' as opposed to unconventional; Jacquee Storozynski-Toll (2011) wrote Vera 'looks like a woman having a menopausal breakdown'; and David W (2011) observes that '[s]eeing Brends continually try to run like a policewoman was ridiculous'. Such responses indicate that there are divergent views about whether Vera is an authentic or realistic depiction of a middle-aged woman. Indeed audiences interpret meanings presented to them in different ways, often according to their own experiences. These discussions illustrate the circulation of tacit knowledge and the ways online audiences, as a collective intelligence, test half formed ideas to ask interpretative questions (cf. Williams, 2009)

However, bloggers aligned with social movement sites, in general, do not have much faith that television will ever offer adequate portrayals. In their identification of stereotypes, social movement bloggers take issue with perceived unrealistic portrayals. For instance, the programme *Drop Dead Diva* is a comedy that features a larger woman in the main role. However, this woman is actually a very thin model killed in a car accident, and brought back to life as an overweight highly intelligent lawyer in search of the meaning of inner beauty as penance for her superficial life. One thread on the *Big Fat Blog*, 'Will Drop Dead Diva Live up to the Hype?', illustrates the fat acceptance movement's scepticism and negativity about depictions of fat people on television. According to Kimdog:

> … this show required a gimmick to get a fat woman center stage … after all, this is the metaphorical 'skinny woman trapped in a fat woman's body' – the mantra of dieting women everywhere. I would much rather see a show where the lead is a fat woman (in a fat woman's body) who is empowered, happy and successful; that would be a true breakthrough (2009).

Many of the bloggers took a similar response – they were 'pretty skeptical' (withoutscene, 2009); not 'hugely impressed' because there were the 'predictable food-obsession jokes with the fat woman character' (MarilynW, 2009); 'no matter what their good intentions are, [mainstream media] will never fully be able to fully embrace size acceptance' (pani113, 2009).

Posters on the *Big Fat Blog* who wrote about the programme *Huge*, a drama about teenagers and staff at a weight loss camp, took a similar stance to discussions about *Drop Dead Diva*. Indiefilmchick sums up what many posters on this site feel about mainstream television media:

> This is going to sound horrible but tv never gets it right. In all the fat women portrayals and FA entertainment projects, they never get it right. Never have I seen my own experiences onscreen (2010).

Similar tendencies can be seen in some disability engagement with storylines of popular television shows such as *Beverly Hills 90210's* treatment of Silver's bipolar diagnosis:

> … they made Silver, one of the primary characters, bipolar, and I had to stop watching. The story arc around her 'mental breakdown' and subsequent hospitalization was so offensive and unrealistic (Abbyjean, 2009).

Prolific disability blogger s.e. smith was just as unimpressed with a *Grey's Anatomy's* storyline regarding the birth of a child with a disability. Although s.e. smith acknowledges that a debate regarding the social devaluing of disability took place throughout the episode, ultimately for s.e. smith:

> The creators seemed to be aiming for a subtext suggesting that disability is not inherently bad and terrible and that disabled people are human beings with rights and autonomy. However, what it actually did was imply that people with disabilities aren't authorities on their own existence (2012).

What these discussions about the desire for realistic portrayals show is that disability, obesity and ageing, while relevant to online audiences and social movements' self-identity, can be subject to disabling social attitudes in particular contexts. As David Gauntlett (2002) argues, media representation will often perpetuate the disempowered position of certain groups by invoking pejorative beliefs. For example, while it is illegal to discriminate on the basis of disability, media images will routinely reinforce negative stereotypes and associations regarding disability. Television typically presents disability, obesity and ageing as clearly defined categories without acknowledging the importance of context and cultural construction. Disability, obesity and ageing, as we argue throughout this book, are context specific.

Quantification

According to Lorenzo-Dus (2009, p. 189), televisual discourse mediates reality through the way it 'reflects and constructs particular values and beliefs about different aspects of "reality"'. Disability, obesity and ageing cannot be definitively defined – these identity categories are always context specific. For example, a recent study into perceptions of ageing in America found that most people associated ageing with an inability to drive or walk up stairs (see Pew Research, 2009). Therefore in an environment without cars and stairs, would ageing mean something different? Likewise, Richardson (2010, p. 75) argues that in situations when the built environment is accessible wheelchair users are not disabled, and he contends that the cultural definition of fat has changed to the point where his students refer to 1950s Hollywood star Marilyn Monroe as a 'big'un'.

Online audiences on both official and viewer-generated sites discuss the way the media tries to quantify or impose identifications as facts, without qualification. For example, participants on *The Biggest Loser* discussion forum frequently debate whether a contestant is 'really fat enough' to participate on *The Biggest Loser.*

Similarly ageing in *Hot in Cleveland* is a contested topic amongst online audiences and in programme reviews because the show's basic premise rests on an unquantifiable definition of old:

> Take three ladies of 'a certain age' (which in LA-speak presumably means pretty much anyone over 35) tired of the vacuous California lifestyle, plonk them down in the mid-west where people actually eat real food as opposed to macrobiotic tofu and hey, presto! A sitcom is born. Basically a remake of The Golden Girls with a dash of Sex and the City (50 – it's the new 30. We've still got it!) (Kelly, 2011).

Even Artie, a character who uses a wheelchair in *Glee*, is not always interpreted as disabled – because he has a good attitude and integrates well with the other students in the school show choir or so-called Glee club:

> Him being in a wheelchair has zero to do with his personality, and as a viewer you don't notice it – and not that the kids didn't care [about the inaccessible environment he must navigate daily] because they loved him. They just never took the time to think how hard being disabled could be because Artie doesn't make it seem so bad after all (Kennedy, 2009).

Similarly, when another *Glee* character – Quinn – became paralyzed following a car accident in Season 3, online audiences debated whether she was 'really disabled' because she was undergoing physiotherapy to learn to walk again with varying degrees of success (Glee Forum, 2012). In a thread on the official *Glee* forum entitled 'How Disabled Does one Have to be Before They are Considered "Disabled"?' a discussion regarding whether disability could be definitively defined was initiated by online audience member jaque_the_ripper (2012) who observed that Quinn had experienced a lot of 'hate' from online audiences because she was '"lying" about being disabled'. For jaque_the_ripper 'Quinn was still very much disabled' despite her progress in physiotherapy, yet Hermione (2012) believed Quinn should be considered injured rather than disabled. These two posters and other online audience members debated the meaning of disability and how Quinn's physical impairment helped to shape hers and other characters. When jaque_the_ripper offered 'having a physical or mental condition that limits movement, senses, or activities' as a definition of disabled, Hermione responded that in that case she would be disabled 'because I need glasses. My sense is limited'. Although television representations may appear to offer definitive categories around disability, obesity and ageing, online audiences disagree as to who in particular fit into these groups.

A particular concern of ours in this book is the way disabling social attitudes are constructed regarding disability, obesity and ageing in media discourse, including both on television and in online forums. A particularly important disabling social attitude is overt prejudice – often reflected in audience criticism of the very presence of images of disability, obesity and ageing on television.

That's Not Something I Want to See!

As we discussed in the previous chapter, disabled, old and obese bodies have long been considered 'unwatchable' because they make audiences feel uncomfortable about the tenuous control they have over their own bodies. For Shakespeare (1994, p. 297), negative attributes are ascribed to non-normative bodies as part of a general strategy of disidentification. Television and other media utilize a 'normative formula' (Snyder & Mitchell, 2010, p. 193) to perpetuate stigma against certain groups and discourage empathy with them. Indeed audiences often seek to deny these aspects of themselves.

When *Mike & Molly* aired in 2010 there was public outrage on online forums at the prospect of two fat characters kissing on television. For example, Arnold Ward (2010) comments ' … grossly fat people are less attractive, get over it'; and NYU Student (2010) said, 'Maybe the tiny minority with a fatty fetish [want to see fat characters on TV] but face facts – the vast majority of us do not. Jiggling, quivering rolls of fat make me nauseous as well … '. Fat people kissing and showing affection was apparently something audiences did not want to see, as expressed by *Marie Claire* writer Maura Kelly:

> I think I'd be grossed out if I had to watch two characters with rolls and rolls of fat kissing each other … because I'd be grossed out if I had to watch them doing anything. To be brutally honest, even in real life, I find it aesthetically displeasing to watch a very, very fat person simply walk across a room – just like I'd find it distressing if I saw a very drunk person stumbling across a bar or a heroine addict slumping in a chair (2010).

The above quote is taken from an article that appeared on *Marie Claire* online. Its author Maura Kelly garnered mainstream media attention as well as responses from online social activists. Most posters chastized the editor of the magazine for publishing the article; and because they considered that Kelly's article was 'insensitive', 'offensive', and 'rude' ('Comments', n.d.) as this indicative comment illustrates:

> What a stupid insensitive idiot you are Ms. Kelly. So only models should be on tv and movies? Can we really deal with tv shows that only have Megan Fox's 'talent'? (Michael Wenthold, 2011).

The *Big Fat Blog* 'Virtual Kiss-In!!!' (2010) was an organized worldwide response to Kelly's *Marie Claire* article. With the aim of contesting and challenging this kind of belief, the fat acceptance movement rallied online uploading hundreds of videos and photographs of themselves kissing their partners, romantic interests, children, and relatives. Thus online forums provided both the opportunity to perpetuate (through the initial article) and question (through the kiss-in) socially disabling attitudes.

Similarly, when Cerrie Burnell began co-hosting the BBC children's network, CBeebies in 2009, several parents took exception to a person with a disability hosting a television show watched by children and posted their complaints on the BBC website. Several postings which claimed the presenter's disability gave their children nightmares were considered inflammatory and were removed from BBC website (Thomas, 2009). Whereas detractors claimed that the BBC had gone overboard in its attempt to include 'minorities', supporters of Burnell and the BBC argued parents were projecting their own prejudices onto children. Online forums therefore provided a vital space for the public to debate these important issues.

In reaction to the reality programme *Hotter Than My Daughter* most online responses to *SodaHead*, the opinion-based community site, found the programme's idea 'disgusting' (ASPEN, 2010; LEXY, 2010; NotWithOutAFight, 2010; Son of Furious, 2010). The programme's underlying assumption is that mother and daughter are competing over who has the best dress sense and overall style; the public judge the contestants about their style before and after their final makeover. Most of the mothers – women generally over 40 – loudly and persistently claim they are more 'physically and sexually attractive' than their daughters (Mangan, 2010). Some contestants are older; for example, 56 year old grandmother Carolene who is the mother of 26 year old Alysha. The subtext of the online posts is that mothers over 40 should dress and act in a more demure way, and not compete with their daughters in terms of beauty, style and sexiness:

> Wow … a show that highlights desperate middle aged women franticly trying to pretend their 40's are their 20's reborn. I feel so sorry for the daughters, it must be terribly embarrassing for them. Madonna's daughter is stunning, the material girl is delusional if she thinks that she can compete even with her daughter being as young as she is (Zoel, 2010).

Here, Zoel states that Madonna is 'delusional', implying that youth is by its very nature sexier than old age – thereby, reiterating televisual media's narrowly defined view of equating sexiness with youthfulness. What the programme and online audience comments do not make clear is when precisely does young become old?

Viewers and fans often use television websites in ways not intended by television programme producers. For instance, viewers can express views very different from networks about participants and characters (Gillan, 2011). For this reason, according to Gillan, television websites can be seen as *excess* by programme makers who know that website forums will spill out despite the network's desire to contain them. In addition to these ongoing critiques about television representations, some audiences may simply go online to discuss their favourite characters and television shows.

I Like This

We have found many examples of discussions about television shows where online audience members engage in an appreciation for the show or specific characters. Furthermore, the strength of audience members' identifications and disidentifications is reflected in online discussions. This engagement is now part of television entertainment. Whereas so called cult television shows such as *Star Trek* have long elicited extraordinary online followings, the availability of television companion websites for almost all television programmes has seen regular viewer websites similarly thrive (Deery, 2003, p. 173). Audience appreciation and engagement after the programme ends is evident on official sites that celebrate the representation of disability, obesity and ageing. For example, *The Voice* Australia relied heavily on tele-participation, including official and unofficial websites and social networking, to maintain a circular flow of audience participation during and after the airing of each show. In the following section we consider the representation of disability, obesity and ageing during the battle round of *The Voice* and the way these images (and meanings) were publicly debated in comments following the YouTube videos of selected performances on *The Voice*'s official YouTube channel.

Case Study: *The Voice*

The Voice is an international television franchise that emphasizes the importance of talent over looks that aired from 15 April to 18 June 2012 on Channel 9 in Australia. A diverse range of contestants competed in the show, including disabled, old(er) and fat performers. In an article entitled 'New Rule: Great Voices Never get old' Andrew Murphett (2012) describes the franchise as 'quirky' citing 9's head of development explanation that the Dutch version included 'a dwarf and two twins'. The final four Australian competitors demonstrate this philosophy. They were (in order of their final placing) Karise Eden, Darren Percival, Rachael Leahcar and Sarah De Bono.

Whereas Sarah could be described as possessing the look required of a pop singer, the other finalists – to a greater or lesser degree – fit the identifications we are concerned with in this book. Aged 40, Darren had struggled to break into the music industry for 22 years and was described as not meeting 'commercial music criteria' (*The Voice*, 2012). Similarly, Karise, although possessing a powerful enough voice to finally win the competition, has a larger body than the conventional commercial singer. Finally, Rachael has vision impairment. These singers were subjected to particular framing techniques and emotional cues related to their looks and back-story as well as their disability, body size and age. *The Voice* relied heavily on social media throughout its two month duration, integrating tweets in the show and encouraging viewers to continue their engagement with the franchise online.

The Voice has three stages of competition – the blind audition, the battle round and live stage shows. Contestants are coached through the series by celebrity mentors Keith Urban, Delta Goodrem, Joel Madden or Seal, who teach them industry secrets to hone their performances and establish themselves as marketable commodities. During the blind auditions, the mentors have their backs to the potential contestants as they audition, turning their chair only if they would like to work with the singer. As such they are privy only to the audience reaction and the singer's voice.

In a semiotic coup, Rachael – an actual blind singer – performed in the blind audition. Channel 9 used this moment in their aggressive marketing of the programme seemingly to demonstrate the importance of talent. Beth Haller argues in the context of the news media that 'people who have visually apparent disabilities are valued ... because of the unspoken visual and emotional cues they provide' (2000, p. 225). Rachael provided such visual and emotional cues in *The Voice*. In addition, her admission that she could not see if anyone had turned their chair registered with the mentors who had just watched the audience immediately rise to a standing ovation; thus the mentors were privy to the emotional cues of disability. When pleading their respective cases, the mentors used emotionally loaded terminology to try to convince Rachael to join their team. Seal described her as courageous, Joel told her she was special, Keith told her she was beautiful, while Delta drew on her own experience of surviving cancer to assure Rachael that on her team it would always be about her voice, not her disability. Rachael chose Delta.

Once the mentors have selected a team of 12, the show progresses to the battle round where the coaches pit two of their team against each other. The two singers perform a duet (or battle) and their coach selects which contestant will go forward to the live stage shows based on that performance. Viewers responded enthusiastically to the producer's call to tele-participation both during and after the on air texts. In addition to 'I like this' discussions, the themes of disability, body size and ageing were explored in the social media discourse. This was especially true during the battle round.

Rachael was overwhelmingly presented as angelic or as what Martin Norden coined a 'sweet innocent' on the programme and in the associated social media discourse (1994, p. 33). Norden describes this characterization as 'invariably a child or young unmarried woman' who is:

> … perfect in every way except for the disability; respectful, humble, gentle, cheerful, godly, pure and exceptionally pitiable … . Typically, the Sweet Innocent was far more reactive than proactive and seemed to bring out the protectiveness of every good-hearted able-bodied person who came his or her way (p. 33).

It is evident that Rachael Leahcar's performance and interactions on *The Voice* embodies Norden's description of the sweet innocent. However, in the YouTube comments, Rachael's success was often attributed to her having a disability. The programme makers can therefore not control what the audience does with the images and discourses they are offered. For instance, the idea that Rachael was advancing in the competition on the basis of her disability rather than talent was a common point of view on YouTube following her battle round video of *Over the Rainbow*, as this comment from Isabela Rivas (2012) demonstrates:

> I'm not saying any of this to be mean, just realistic; Adam has a stronger voice. Rachel has a sad story and good control, sure. But I think Adam was better. I don't think it would've mattered what he'd done on the night, because in the end, they've built this show up using Rachel and her story. They set Adam up to get knocked off in this round.

Whereas Rachael's disability was constantly mentioned in the advertising for *The Voice*, so too was the large number of contestants who did not fit the conventional image of a pop singer by virtue of age or body size. For example, several singers who are considered old or ageing in the music industry competed successfully in the auditions.

Darren was amongst several ageing performers, some of whom were described on the show as 'ageing rockers'. Following Darren's battle against a much younger singer, mentor Keith Urban asked Darren why he (Keith) should choose him, making explicit reference to Darren's age and asking him why this opportunity would be different at this time of his life. The YouTube comments following this video also made frequent reference to Darren's age. However, unlike the comments discussing Rachael, the discourse about Darren accepted the show's vision of the world – thus, reinforcing the symbolic power of the programme that with the right attitude, and makeover, age should be no barrier. Commenters accepted the notion that talent was more important than age:

> I prefer Darren's voice. The rasp ages the lyric, making it seem to be words of wisdom from an old man. The song itself is beautiful and arrived at a point when it was needed in my life. I thank the producers of the show for organizing its release and re-introducing a classic to the general (GarySharp, 2012).

> Some people think he's not marketable but I do not care, I'll vote for him (20Valvetop, 2012).

Thus the online audience accepted the claims made explicit in the programme – that age was not a barrier, that age adds wisdom and that success in the music industry is related to both talent and image creation. Karise Eden battled Paula who also challenges the conventionally accepted body size in the music industry. However, the YouTube audience was surprisingly moot about their appearance, focusing instead on talent, often alluding to Karise's 'huge' future in the music industry or her 'massive' voice. In these conversations synonyms associated with weight were repurposed as positive attributes.

The programme was explicit in the vision of the world it was attempting to promote and aggressively used overflow and a multiplatform to encourage tele-participation. Analysis of the comments following the YouTube videos of the battle rounds, when favoured contestants progressed through to the real competition, demonstrate that viewers of *The Voice* appear to have accepted its vision of the world.

Conclusion

Along with television itself, television websites and popular culture blogs are now a major medium in (re)presenting disability, obesity and ageing. The television industry can make certain perspectives and images visible – it has the symbolic power to influence and shape the minds of ordinary viewers (Couldry, 2000). However, increasingly, online spaces provide a platform for television viewers to contest this symbolic power and dominant discourses of disability, obesity and ageing. Although this is especially so for activist groups, other unofficial and official forums also provide spaces for contestation.

Official-generated and viewer-generated websites (including the disability and fat acceptance movements' online forums) have multiplied – in unprecedented ways. Part of this proliferation can be attributed to the audience's ability and power to contest media representations. The online audiences and social movements are active and vocal about what is presented on mainstream television. As a result of the read–write web, audiences and viewers can now instantly comment, criticize and censor the symbolic forms used by programme makers. Audiences and viewers actually respond in mixed and varied ways. Underlying their responses is the degree to which individuals and audiences identify with characters or ordinary people who participate on television.

Although the media discourse produced by the television institutions circulates, viewers and audiences level of engagement varies on television's official-generated and viewer-generated websites. From these responses and the four themes identified, we recognize that viewers do more than just 'decoding' the 'encoding' of media messages in oppositional, preferred and negotiated ways as Hall (1980, pp. 47–49) outlined in his pioneering work. Viewers and audiences, especially those mobilized within fat acceptance and disability movements, create counter examples to contest and challenge socially disabling beliefs. In the following chapter, we focus on whether audiences identify or disidentify with the depictions presented in television programmes.

Chapter 4
Audience Activity: Identification, Disidentification and Online Activity

> My 95 year old father has been watching Grumpy Old Men, and reckons those young pups don't have too much they can complain about. He actually got pretty grumpy about it, too! (73yearsyoung, 2005).

> In some ways fat bodies are our current culture's dumping ground for fear and loathing: we are the go-to places for thrashing out anxiety about consumption and excess, death and disease, work ethic and individual responsibility, boundaries and restraint, ugliness and beauty. Fat bodies are politicised – even politicians literally use fat as short-hand for bad, wrong, excessive. Fat bodies are ridiculed, dehumanised, demonised and charged with meaning (My Milk Spilt, 2011).

This chapter surveys the way online audiences watch and interpret television texts, with a particular focus on disability, obesity and ageing as identification targets. Within broadcast media, online forums (official and unofficial) enable and produce connections between identity categories and audience identifications of disabled, obese and old. Online audiences like 73yearsyoung and My Milk Spilt quoted above draw on representations within programmes, as well as what they read about in magazines, newspapers, and social media such as Facebook and Twitter. In addition, audiences talk about these representations online and undoubtedly with co-workers, family, and friends. Online audience members engage in a nuanced way and often negotiate the preferred meanings offered in media representations.

We do not assess *active audiences* in this book; rather, we examine audiences' activities online to gain insight into the negotiation of media messages. Audience activity, for Costello and Moore (2007, p. 132), is expressed as a continuous series of activities that are apparent in various interactive comings and goings on the Internet. In response to discourses of disability, obesity and ageing represented on television, we are concerned with two types of audience activity:

- identification with the characters in the programme; and
- online tele-participation during and after the programme.

Television programmes and their accompanying websites, according to Gray, offer identities that viewers and online audiences can grapple with (Gray, 2008, p. 121). Williams (2009, p. 58) takes the similar view that individuals put popular culture to use in such a way that they can perform their social identity and establish community. The attraction to any particular television website activity – be it *Glee, The Biggest Loser* or *Grumpy Old* – cannot be divorced from how individuals conceive of their identities (p. 58). Many online audience members participate on official-generated or unofficial-generated sites because they identify with the disabled or obese or old(er) bodies represented on television.

Although televisual media attempts to essentialize characters' identities – especially those who have fat, old and disabled bodies – televisual media and audiences do not necessarily concur in their responses to key questions such as What *is* old age? What *is* obese? What *is* disability? Television aims to quantify disability, obesity and age, without acknowledging the ways these identities are culturally and contextually constructed and changeable. For example, in shows such as *The Biggest Loser,* bodies are situated as obese as if that is a fact. This conception is rarely perceived as a sub-conscious and uncontested cultural and medical belief about large-sized bodies. Likewise, in *10 Years Younger in 10 Days,* ageing is presented as a lifestyle choice or a state of mind. Similarly, characters with disability in many primetime programmes are frequently constructed as having a good or a bad attitude in ways that do not recognize the social construction of disability. For instance, the character Jason Street in *Friday Night Lights* was constructed in different ways depending on his attitude. When his family sued the school to pay for physiotherapy and adaptations to their home following Jason's football injury that caused paralysis to his lower body the community believed he was exhibiting a bad attitude. However, throughout the majority of the series Jason had a good attitude because he got on with his life. Similarly, participants on *Extreme Makeover* are constructed as worthy recipients of charity because of their positive attitude in spite of their disability.

Disabled, old and obese characters have historically been little more than peripheral characters used for semiotic shorthand. More recently, however, these characters have been given leading roles on popular primetime television in shows such as *Friday Night Lights*, *The West Wing*, *Mike & Molly*, *Hot in Cleveland* and *Everybody Loves Raymond.* Television's search for essentialist identities continues despite this increasingly diverse range of representations.

This chapter considers the way television media is defining identity categories such as disabled, fat and old, and the immediate and direct responses of online audiences to what they are seeing. We begin with an interrogation of the way Western audiences participate in television websites in the context of broader critiques of audience and reception. As discussed in the previous chapter, television is now subject to overflow, and audiences engage in tele-participation in ways that both question and reinforce the vision of the world offered on television. The chapter then moves to consider the emotional phenomenon described by Jonathan Cohen as identification. For Cohen (2001), identifying with characters or participants often occurs when audiences share or have loved ones with the same characteristics, interests, affinities and experiences. We divide the scholarship into two sets of responses – identification and disidentification. Both responses belong to the same emotional realm and audience members may oscillate between the two. Television producers actively encourage audiences to either identify or disidentify with certain characters in programmes through stylistic techniques such as editing, framing, casting and music.

The chapter finishes with a case study discussion of Selena Brown, a contestant with a disability on *The Biggest Loser: Singles* (2012) – the focus is on how the programme persists in stigmatising individuals as a leverage to attract audiences. Online audiences either relate to, or feel for Selena or they find her objectionable. We contend that television programmes like *The Biggest Loser* perpetuate stigma against certain individuals and discourage empathy with them through their production style and techniques. However, as we outline in the following section, audiences are not passive – they negotiate the meanings presented to them on television.

Audiences who Participate in Television Websites

Although audiences are recognized within cultural and media studies as having choice and of interpreting television texts through their own experiences and contexts, audiences may still, in some circumstances, accept the preferred media message. For example, as discussed in the previous chapter, when *Glee*'s series regular character with a disability Artie was afforded a typical 'inspirational cripple' storyline different online audiences interpreted the construction in different ways. For television reviewers dos Santos (2009) and Kennedy (2009), the messages were empowering whereas disability bloggers criticized the use of this common stereotype (s.e. smith, 2009; wheelchair dancer, 2009).

As we discussed in Chapter 2, much of the online discussion focuses on interpretative questions whereby online audience members test ideas, debate concepts and draw on each other's experiences to consider the issues as a form of 'collective intelligence' (cf. Williams, 2009). Thus, people do more than decode texts according to their own contexts – they now also draw on other people's contexts through the interpretative questions discussed online.

Interpretative questions seldom have correct answers – often questions such as these can be answered with supporting evidence from the television text and can have several answers, which are assessed by forum members. Many of the interpretative questions on online television forums deal with the themes we outlined in the previous chapter, such as stereotypes, realism, quantification, disgust and affinity. For instance on *The Biggest Loser* (2012) unofficial *Whirlpool* site discussants asked interpretative questions about quantification:

> Is it just me or are some of the contestants on this year's show not really that big? (mrmister, 2012).
>
> As I recall Jonny Depp's character in that movie wasn't fat. So how does that fit with your enabler model? (june27, 2012).

These questions and the response to them reveal how creating meaning about identity categories such as disability, obesity and ageing is visible, observable and communal. The online forums provide space and opportunities for anybody to participate in the discourse. Thus online forums hold an important position within the experience of viewing television, especially in the formation of communities of interest.

Susan Boyle: Responses from One Community of Interest

One such community of interest emerged in association with *Britain's Got Talent* contestant Susan Boyle. To some extent, Susan Boyle embodies all of the identities – that is, disabled, overweight, and ageing – we are concerned with in this book. The audience response to her story offers an insight into audience activity. When Susan Boyle first took to the stage to audition for *Britain's Got Talent* in 2009, the studio audience was unwelcoming. Her frumpy appearance was juxtaposed with a close-up of a young attractive girl in the audience scoffing when Susan Boyle described her dream of becoming a professional singer. As an unattractive, slightly overweight, 47-year-old woman with bushy eyebrows, her image was not at all conducive to that of a professional singer. The crowd immediately knew how to react to Boyle – laugh. The judges, likewise, expressed scepticism.

Television audiences, who are familiar with the audition on talent programmes such as *Britain's Got Talent*, know that the television producers orchestrate the audition to engender emotion from the audience. In talent programmes like *Britain's Got Talent,* audiences barrack for who gets through to the finals. This affect is evident in the mixture of hesitation, surprise and applause shown by the audience and the judges to Susan Boyle's performance. Middle-aged women like Boyle are often stereotyped as frumpy, asexual, and passive in television texts. The crowd's instantaneous reaction to Boyle's appearance reveals how programme makers use the audience's tacit knowledge – in this case about middle-aged female identity – and the elements that make up talent shows.

When Susan Boyle begins singing, however, the judges and audience begin to participate in a different narrative – suddenly Susan is *inspirational,* her singing talent is more impressive because she is unattractive, unknown, and an unlikely idol.

Later, various profiles, documentaries and new reports, revealed that Susan also had a disability. Online activity on her official website immediately after her appearance on *Britain's Got Talent* demonstrates the ways disability, obesity and ageing can be something audiences identify with and/or reject as part of their viewing experience. Ultimately, many ordinary viewers empathize with Susan Boyle because they also felt fat, old and disabled, as the following post suggests:

> The more I play her video and listen to her singing, the more I grow to admire this most unassuming lady. Susan is the model and heroine of the normal masses … the majority of us who have ordinary lives, doing ordinary things and may be old, disabled, unemployed, fat, etc. … She brings hope and light. What a lady! (ngayonatkailanman, 2009).

Middle-aged women such as Boyle are disadvantaged in Western countries by existing 'codes of celebrity' – rooted in sexist and ageist ways of thinking – which value youthful, able and slim bodies (Negra & Holmes cited in Holmes, 2010, p. 75). This was recognized by online audiences, as demonstrated by Claire's critique:

> It almost feels as if people are saying 'It's wrong that such a beautiful voice comes from such ordinary looking woman'. I'm not going to lie and say that I think she's conventionaly beautiful. She's not … but it's just disheartening that the selling point isn't her voice (which is amazing) it's that this magical voice belongs to HER (2009).

Although the media constructed Susan Boyle as old, fat and disabled, none of these categories is quantifiable as such – attesting to what is old, fat and disabled is bounded by the context in which these identities are situated. The mediated characterisations television offers are both too narrow and too extreme (Andrejevic, 2004; Turner, 2009). However, as the post responses above indicate, the televisual media cannot harness online audience responses to shore up their essentialist depictions. One reason this divergence occurs is that audiences interpret from their own experience and bring their tacit knowledge and reading of other texts to their online forum discussions (Livingstone, 2005; Williams, 2009, p. 42). For example, as expressed by ngayonatkailanman, we have all felt inadequate (or disabled, old and fat) at some point, whereas Claire questions the conflation of looks with talent. These two comments acknowledge important points about the contexts in which disability, obesity and ageing are judged and the way television attempts to quantify these.

Although most people engaging with the media today are often aware of media techniques, many do not always know how the symbolic power of the media works. Some audiences are oblivious to television's business activities and the necessity to question the power of the media (Couldry, 2000; Lotz, 2007). Yet others make choices and audiences take pleasure in what is presented without necessarily accepting or taking on board the preferred views of a television programme (Gauntlett, 2002, p. 17; Rayner, Wall, & Kruger, 2004, p. 97).

In the next section we contextualize the process Cohen (2001) describes as 'identification'. Our discussion reiterates Hall's (1980) framework of encoding/decoding in the sense that television production encodes a preferred message, but online audiences (and audiences in general) do not necessarily decode the message in the way framed by the media – yet often they do.

Identification and Television Online Audience

According to Godlewski and Perse (2010), producers use technical features, emotive influences and programme websites to shape sympathetic or unsympathetic audience responses towards certain characters. *Technical features* comprise repetition of content, camera angles, music and use of close-ups. *Emotive influences* are created through the choice of music, dialogue and casting. Finally, additional exposure and repetition are conveyed through the *programme websites*. These three features combined work to create a rapport between online audiences and on air characters and participants.

Rapport with media characters in all kinds of television programming is essential to getting viewers involved in the programme (Godlewski & Perse, 2010, p. 151; see also Eyal & Rubin, 2003). Identification with media characters is a topic that traverses many areas of media and cultural studies, including film studies, media psychology and television entertainment. Judith Butler makes two significant points about the process of identification and disidentification in her work (cited in Fuss, 1995, p. 7) First, Butler proposes that while it may appear that an individual is refusing to identify with another, it might be more accurate to say that the act of identifying 'has already been made and denied in the unconscious' (p. 7). Second, Butler claims that 'identifications are never brought to full closure' – often they 'are vehicles' for another identification (p. 6). But, ultimately, identifications fail to be fully realized (p. 6). Indeed Butler's contribution goes some way to explaining why some online audiences – who share a similar identity position – may disidentify with characters or participants.

Television draws on stereotypes to represent minority groups in such a way that they become archetypes and shape social reality (Gray, 2008). As Major, Spencer, Schmader, Wolfe, & Crocker (1998) argue, stereotypical representations of particular groups perpetuate stigma against them. These images then become culturally recognizable messages that may impact on whether people identify as being part of this group (Major et al.). For instance, disability representations can evoke emotion 'to cement longstanding associations of stigma with bodily difference' (Snyder & Mitchell, 2010, p. 192). As a result, people with disability seek to disassociate (Major et al., 1998) with televisual representations of disability in the way Butler describes above. Similarly people who are obese and old may seek to disassociate from a character's traits even though it is similar to their own. For instance, posters on the *Big Fat Blog* frequently disassociate themselves from characters on primetime television programmes who are obese because those characters do not accept their size. For the *Big Fat Blog* posters it's about attitude. The *Big Fat Blog* discussants consider *The Biggest Loser* programme as having the wrong attitude just as *The Biggest Loser* trainers see the obese contestants as having the wrong attitude. A few older audience members did not connect with frumpy, ageing middle-aged characters on the programme *Vera* – as some of their comments, cited in the previous chapter, illustrate. We surmise that these online audiences found the character Vera too matronly and unpolished.

Jonathon Cohen (2001) argues that the moment of identifying occurs when a viewer shares a character's perspective, and vicariously begins to participate in the experiences of that character (p. 249). However, the actual process of identifying is filtered through the viewer's experience and world view (Cohen 2006, p. 185). Even though online audiences write about their response to contestants such as Susan Boyle, we concur with Cohen (2001, p. 249) that these comments are representative of a moment in time – generally while the programme is aired or while the website is accessible. Although online conversations are just as fleeting as water-cooler conversations, they are perhaps more significant and worthy of analysis because they too form a cultural text that others can access. And moreover online conversations in their written interpretation of the television text offer examples of global responses to televisual texts.

Of course some viewers perceive themselves to be like a character when they actually aren't (Chory-Assad & Yanen, 2005; Hoffner & Buchanan, 2005). According to Hoffner and Buchanan (p. 342), when people believe they are similar to characters, or aspire to have characters' qualities, these viewers tend to participate in 'wishful identification'. This may help to explain why older people distance themselves from images of old people on television – their preference is for youthful looking older people as they would like to be. Images that celebrate the ability to deny the physical signs of ageing simultaneously achieve two things – they liberate older people from traditional stereotypes of ageing as being unattractive and undesirable, and at the same time this liberation ties older people to desiring a youthful body, a task that is ultimately unachievable for most.

Identifying as Old

From Krout's (cited in Fishman, 2010, p. 48) perspective, baby boomers do not want to appear old, nor do they 'identify with those older than themselves'. This is a reoccurring storyline in the sitcom *Hot in Cleveland* in which the characters both disavow the process of ageing and approximate youthful qualities. Similarly, Krout makes a broad claim that baby boomers prefer 'to think that they can remain youthful – or at least not become old' (cited in Fishman, p. 48). In our example of older viewers who refuse to identify with older characters or participants – often claiming that this is 'not' 'me' – at some level the action of identitifying 'has already taken place' (Butler, 1993, p. 113). Thus, their response upholds Butler's position that 'disidentification is part of the common practice of identification itself' (2004, pp. 145–146).

Grumpiness or disgruntlement is constructed as a symptom of old age in the *Grumpy Old Men* and *Grumpy Old Women* television series and programmes such as *One Foot in the Grave.* On television being too old is constructed as a personal affliction, thus, ageing (rather than ageism) is presented as problematic. The problem is ageing itself that manifests itself in the attitude of grumpiness. However, the *Grumpy Old Men* and *Grumpy Old Women* television series celebrates grumpiness, the series equates grumpiness with a particular sociocultural construction of midlife. The grumpiness brand extends the overflow of the televisual beyond the television series to companion books and other merchandise, and online forums such as *Grumpier Old Men* and *GoodOldTalk.com* (see 'Grumpy Old Men and Grumpy Old Women' thread). Thereby it expands the mediated space in which to explore midlife grumpiness. Participants on these forums, many of whom declare they are no longer young, explicitly align grumpiness with growing older, so their public declarations of irritability reveals grumpiness to be both an identifier of older age and an act of identifying (Cohen, 2001):

> Love this show, although I never cease to be horrified by how much I identify with all the grumpiness. (PS – I do wish they'd show more of Germaine, but that's me being grumpy I suppose) (iorarua ®, 2010).

Terms such as the 'young–old', and the 'near–elderly', which are typically applied to baby boomers (Gullette, 2011, p. 9), create the impression of dwindling youth. Yet baby boomers tend to resist old age stereotypes (Fishman, 2010, p. 48). As a programme, *Grumpy Old* opens a space to reclaim old age stereotypes, and simultaneously makes it possible for online viewers to converse about how they identify and disidentify with being old. As one online viewer points out, those old people featured on the show are not me:

> I don't think of myself as one (in fact I still think of myself as 25 years old, but that's another story), but I can't help but sympathise with some of the comments (73yearsyoung, 2005).

Identifying as Obese

Although online audiences may recognize and critique the limited characterizations of disability, obesity and ageing available on television, often what they disidentify with is ostensibly bad attitudes. For example, in the case of the *Biggest Loser* online, many audiences identify with contestants who are fat, but detest contestants who lack commitment, motivation and focus – namely, those who are content to remain obese. Rarely do audiences on online forums remain distant or detached from participants. Although most online audience posters identify or disidentify with particular participants on *The Biggest Loser* forum, they are likely to spurn television characters who are constructed as choosing to remain disabled, obese and old through their bad attitudes.

In *The Biggest Loser*, the online audience's identification with certain individual contestants is noticeable on the online forums. In particular, audience members appreciate the challenge, self-denial, responsibility, discipline, determination, and techniques the participants display in order to lose weight. However, the obese body itself remains despised and loathed – disavowed by the audience. As will be discussed in Chapter 6, this raises the question of whether it is the slim person inside – rather than the reviled large body – that the online audiences identify with. This idea of identifying with the slim person within is greatly encouraged by the trainers on the programme.

Cohen (2001, p. 261) reiterates Hall's (1980) perspective on decoding that the boost in audience involvement in the message reduces the audience's propensity to critically appraise the programme content. Yet, the discussion of *The Biggest Loser: Singles* (2012) contestant Margie on the official programme website demonstrates that online audiences are often aware of programme makers' editing techniques, and, as a consequence, audience members negotiate the preferred message offered by the producers. Eventual season winner Margie – an outspoken contestant who identifies as lesbian – is constructed as both a bully and a contestant with the right mental attitude on the programme. In a discussion about the way Margie judges the other contestants' efforts on the show, incywebb pointed out the way the audience was being manipulated:

> We really shouldn't make up reasons to dislike these people – the BL editors are already doing their best to warp our impressions into the mould they've pre-determined for the contestants (2012).

Nonetheless forum posters are divided about how much the editing in the programme constructs a participant and how much of the participants' real persona comes forth.

The Biggest Loser: Singles series depicts Margie as having tantrums or hissy fits about the other contestants' behaviour, especially contestants that she considers do not train hard enough. Jacinta gal's and Cupcakewa's comments about Margie's behaviour in Episodes 43 and 44 represent the position that viewers see the real Margie – 'Margie has displayed enough of herself to show that she is emotionally immature. They can't "edit" a character if the person never behaves in that way' (Jacinta gal, 2012a). Similarly, Cupcakewa took the view, 'I found Margie's response disrespectful and probably a real and true insight into her off camera personality' (2012). The idea that Margie is morally questionable – a common fat stereotype – is taken up in the online discussion, despite the recognition that this response was being manipulated by the producers of *The Biggest Loser* through editing, pre-determined characterizations and casting tropes.

Programmes that highlight everyday life issues such as health, relationships and family often tap into viewers' emotions in order to prompt identification with participants (Gray, 2008, p. 121). This televisual device is particularly utilized with characters that televisual audiences would generally view as 'odd' or too 'different' (p. 121). For de Swaan (1997, p. 110), an affective response by an audience member to a character or participant in a programme occurs when individuals emotionally identify '*with*' or disidentify '*from* other people'. He adds that, whether viewers are identifying or disidentifying, this is an affective response that is part of the process of 'identification *of* the others' (p. 110). To identify others de Swaan notes that the 'affective and moral categories' are informed by the faculty of knowing – in other words, conceiving and perceiving what kind of participant is being presented (1997, p. 110). Often this knowing takes the form of tacit knowledge. For this reason, we argue, when ordinary people participate in television programmes such as *The Biggest Loser* and *10 Years Younger in 10 Days,* they are often used to invoke *affect* (Kavka, 2008) and rely on pre-existing normative principles.

Affect

Kavka defines affect 'as material' that is emotions and feelings that 'matters' (2008, p. 33) – here she foregrounds how affect is a mark of reality television because of its significance to the audience. As Kavka (p. 33) explains 'matters' can be defined in a double sense – on the one hand, it relates to the corporeal, on the other, it relates to the senses, as well as producing sensation. Recent writing on reality television explains how this type of programming invokes reactions and displays of emotion from the contestants as well as the audience – the programming is significant to the audiences because viewers can react viscerally (Kavka, 2008; Sender, 2012, p. 21; Skeggs & Wood, 2012). Thus we take Kavka's use of affect to explain how identifications and disidentifications with disability, obesity and ageing (discussed throughout this book) are visceral – that is to say, often materializing through the audience's senses, use of tacit knowledge and bodily responses.

Affect goes some way to explain why online viewers react with emotion towards particular contestants on reality programmes such as *Britain's Got Talent*. In their audience research Skeggs and Wood (2012, p. 6) use the term emotion to reveal how affect is translated into an idea – namely, that when individual feeling (that is, being affected) is changed and fastened to an idea, such as fear, disgust, loathing, joy or elation. Online responses to Susan Boyle's performance, for instance, led us to recognize a specific affective reaction from this audience.

Social movement sites, such as *FWD* or the *Big Fat Blog*, are acutely aware of the way television attempts to invoke affect through constructing certain bodies. For this reason, participants on the *Big Fat Blog* do not identify with *The Biggest Loser* or any of the participants – it is the most despised television programme on this blog. DebraSY epitomizes the view held by most members of the fat acceptance movement:

> And her comments about the Biggest Loser program being about people getting control of their health through diet and exercise? Good Lord. You haven't watched the show recently, have you? It gets worse and worse every season. The last time I saw it they had a segment, I think was called 'the final push', where the contestants exercised until some of them barfed. And, oh, the response to those who had the gall to exercise reasonably, with smiles on their faces, for example. The camera zoomed in on the scornful faces of their trainers. It was clear that this was NOT acceptable (2008).

Affect can be used by programme makers to either create rapport or to create loathing – apparently many *Big Fat Blog* online audiences experience the latter. DebraSY offered an oppositional reading because for her the technical features of the programme promoted this narrative as inspirational through camera framing and music.

As explained by Elsbach and Bhattacharya (2001) and Butler (2004), when viewers disidentify from characteristics or body types similar to themselves, this is part of the act of identifying. Elsbach and Bhattacharya (p. 399), claim that audiences' rejection of those like themselves, is 'cognitive distancing' – to be specific audiences detach from characters or participants who perturb them. Audiences could be disconcerted by the characters' disability, or by their body-size, or by how old they look. For Butler (pp. 145–146), disidentifying can be explained as a 'disavowal', in other words, a desire to dissociate from similar attributes. Audiences often perceive that the identity of a disabled, fat or old character is too different from those considered to be the standard body type – specifically, the norm by which all individuals are measured. Thus, they reject this identity even if they themselves resemble it!

The process of identification and disidentification is essential to the audience activity of negotiating obesity, disability and ageing depictions – negotiating could involve seeking out, confirming, contesting and reshaping true and untrue versions. To borrow from Gray (2008, p. 121), in our analysis of any programmes that depict disability, obesity and old age we ask does the programme encourage online audiences 'to seek out reality'? Or does it persuade audiences to perpetuate polarising opposites such as 'more "thems" that can be contrasted with "us"'? This is especially relevant to obesity, disability and ageing which can only ever be context specific. Online audiences responses to official forum reactions to Selena Brown a participant in *The Biggest Loser* (2012), reveal the ways audiences can be persuaded to perpetuate polarizing opposites when others elect to seek out reality by explaining her hearing impairment and the disabling impact of *The Biggest Loser* regime.

Case Study: *The Biggest Loser: Singles* – Selena

The 2012 Australian series of *The Biggest Loser: Singles* (2012) format focuses on singles looking for romantic love. The series consists of a host Hayley Lewis, and four trainers, Michelle Bridges, Shannan Ponton, Steve Willis (The Commando) and Tiffany Hall. In Episode 1 (2012), programme makers describe contestants as 'unified in their desire to change their lives', and find someone to share their lives with.

The first episode in Series 7 was aired on Channel Ten on 23 January 2012 and the final episode on 8 May 2012. This particular series consisted of 72 episodes. Undoubtedly, part of the programme's construction is to select contestants that a broad range of viewers can identify with. For instance, online audiences are likely to both identify and disidentify with each of the 16 contestants at the start of the series. The competing singles include Margie, Alex, Kasey, Brenda, Rebekah, Graham, Lydia, Michelle, Lisa, Simon, Selena, Hamish, Luke, Ryan, Shane and James. In addition, the contestants' ages range from 20 to 50 years.

Selena Brown is a 21-year-old Indigenous participant from Darwin in the Northern Territory Australia. During the 2012 season Selena was a student studying midwifery at university. Her profile on the Channel Ten official site states that Selena is single and has 'never been in love' ('Contestants', 2012). The official profile also includes a statement from Selena, 'Just because I have a disability doesn't mean I can't achieve my goals and dreams'.

Disidentifying as Disabled

Many online audience members remark that some participants in a programme are planted there by producers to be provocative. Indeed, this could also be true of online posters who troll forums to elicit the reaction of other posters. Producers often choose contestants that most of the audience will disidentify with to increase online audience activity. A case in point is Selena in the *The Biggest Loser: Singles* (2012). Selena has a hearing impairment and was constructed in the programme as having an attitude problem, of using her disability as an excuse to drop out of life. Barnes (1992, p. 14) describes this stereotype as the person with disability being their 'own worst and only enemy' and sees this as a common stereotype of disability on television. These characters are scripted to be able to 'overcome' their 'disability' if they could just stop pitying themselves; however, for most of the programme they just cannot 'rise to the challenge' (Barnes, 1992, p. 14). The construction of this stereotype can be clearly seen in the way the impaired body interacts with the stylistic devices available to the producer (Ellis, 2008).

For instance, audience members are invited to identify with specific participants through the music in the programme. *The Biggest Loser* uses stock music for melodrama. The music initiates 'the viewer's process of identification with the specific show, quickly telling viewers what is going on and where the action takes place' (Granade, 2011, p. 624). Throughout *The Biggest Loser* music is used to emotionally *hail* the viewer to identify with participants. Music is up tempo to create drama when contestants go to weigh-in or start a challenge. Soft piano music is used when contestants talk about their feelings – often to their trainer, or at elimination or at weigh-in (especially when contestants talk about losing weight for their loved ones). The same music is used when contestants, such as Hamish and Michelle, spoke about their budding romance. Soft piano music was especially noticeable when Selena was on camera because she openly expressed feelings more than the other contestants – mainly about being bullied, missing her family and navigating her weight loss journey.

As mentioned above, some online audience members oscillate between identifying and disidentifying with contestants, characters or participants. In Hall's (1980) sense, this could be considered an example of audience members negotiating with the content of the televisual text. For example, in *The Biggest Loser*, Selena is constructed as lacking in motivation, mental stamina and emotional maturity – as well as not having a good work ethic nor being a team player. On three threads devoted to Selena on the *Biggest Loser* discussion forum – 'Selena the Actress', 'Selena Lost 700 Grams in 4 Weeks Outside' and on 'Selena's Bombshell' – posters said that Selena was immature, 'not motivated', 'mentally doesn't get it', 'puts in minimal effort', 'lacks commitment', had a poor 'work ethic', is an actress, 'quits' easily, 'makes excuses', has too many issues (health, disability), and 'never felt included in her team'.

Despite being given two chances to re-enter the show following elimination, Selena appeared as her 'own worst and only enemy' (cf. Barnes, 1992) by not taking full advantage of them. On one occasion she 'eliminated' herself and on another she declined the opportunity to re-enter the competition upon completion of a boot camp with trainer Shannan. When declining the opportunity to re-enter occurred, the discussion forum debated her attitude. The general consensus was that Selena was lazy – she was sabotaging herself and being ungrateful for the opportunity to change her life through *The Biggest Loser*. On *The Biggest Loser: Singles* discussion thread, 'Selena's Bombshell', Jacinta gal (below) oscillates between identifying with the participant Selena's world view and with the online audience's standpoint:

> People have real lives with commitments outside of BL, she doesn't want to miss a whole semester of uni for one week back at BL.
>
> I also don't think she wants to go back into BL as she knows the other contestants are not too fond of her and she lacks motivation – much like Ryan. However, she has been given some tools now and who knows she might maintain her weight loss to date and possibly lose a bit more if she keeps it up. Prior to entering the house she had no tools and didn't know how to train, nor was her mindset even in the slightest altered. At least now she has some idea.
>
> Why did she bother in the first place? Probably because she seriously needs to lose weight and thought it was the way for her. You don't know if you will take to something unless you try it. […] I'm not a Selena fan, she frustrated me and to be honest I will be surprised if she continues her weight loss but hopefully she will prove us all wrong (2012b).

By comparison, The Songbird (below), another forum member clearly disidentified with Selena as a character in the programme. The Songbird (2012) takes issue with the way Selena's disability was presented as part of making excuses. Many posters tend to repeat the mantras of the trainers that 'making excuses' is unacceptable behaviour (georgiegirl66, 2012; the *Whirlpool* forum). Those who continue to make excuses, such as Selena, are considered to be untrainable by *The Biggest Loser* trainers, contestants and forum posters. The Songbird states:

> I bet she walks before she is shown to be the slacker/Non Team Player/Excuse Making creature she is.. Disability aside she is capable of doing great things.. but as long as she keeps saying 'I have a disability'. She is not going to do anything.

> I live with a person who is Hearing Impaired. When Watching Selena earlier on in the Game My partner used to get really frustrated with Selena … especially when she use to turn her hearing aid off rather than listen to her Team … She used to run away to her own little world of silence rather than deal with reality … and Frankly … as my partner said … and I agree 100%. … That is flocking Rude as Hell and won't help her in the Game … and it didn't … (2012).

Identifying with Selena

However, not all posters on the forum disassociate from Selena. Other posters on these same threads go *against* the programme makers' depiction of her character to empathize with her:

> BL may not the way for her [Selena]- she won't be the first or last person to not lose weight the BL way.. indeed how many actually kept it off- BL or any other way for that matter??? She applied, was accepted and so far not going well … who knows if someone else HAD got in how they would have gone … hindsight is 20/20 … I wish her well what-ever happens. (KazbahKaren, 2012).

> Her deafness would alienate her from any social setting (as does mine). Just trying to understand the flow of conversation in any group situation is extremely taxing and sharing a room with 3 other contestants and not being able to keep up with their banter would have filled her with dread. As the saying goes … 'Walk a mile in her shoes … '. (DazzleMe, 2012).

> Selena's bombshell is hardly surprising. She didn't get any support from her team, and most of the time it seemed like they were bullying her. I think her decision to leave the competition was justified (Stillyanos, 2012).

One online poster explains to others on 'Selena's Bombshell' thread the reality of living in the Biggest Loser camp and the pressure to lose weight on national television:

> I don't think anyone could be called lazy for not keeping up with what looks to be a pretty punishing program. I also don't agree with the idea that she took someone else, more deserving's place. No-one would have any idea what an experience like that is really like and what might seem a romantic idea when considered from your loungeroom is not necessarily going to be once you are in amongst it. None of us could really predict how we would react under that type of pressure (criketer, 2012).

Other posters moved between identifying and disidenfying with Selena's position within the programme. In one sense these posters accepted the programme's construction of Selena; however, they also found themselves negotiating the depictions presented by programme makers:

> Selena was never accepted by her team members and other contestants. She must have felt very isolated. I was sad to see her go, and am not convinced she will succeed on the outside losing her weight, but where she is right now it was the right decision. There is nothing to be achieved when you are miserable and have no support. She comes from a totally different environment to the others. I liked the way she explained her decision and stood her ground when Haley and Tiff tried to persuade her otherwise. I hope she is going to be ok (chocifan, 2012).

As can be seen from above, many forum posters empathize with Selena – in particular identifying with her situation – and as a consequence depart from the programme's depictions. Even those who negotiate with the televisual depictions show some empathy towards Selena. In addition, the online posts provide the opportunity to discuss important social issues such as bullying in the wider broadcast media. Callers to talkback radio (Radio National, ABC Australia) claimed to identify with Selena because they too had experienced bullying.

As Gray (2008) argues, analysis of what people do with the unreal, on television, allows us to understand the real. Online audience use of official and unofficial forums, social movement sites, talkback radio, Facebook and blogger sites – enable viewers to contest and challenge televisual experiences. Online audiences in their use of various media forums question the fictions and untruths presented on television programmes to give nuanced responses to the programmes. In the case of Selena (above), some of the online audience contest the televisual portrayal of Selena's disability, of her persona and of her being bullied.

The online discussion of Selena's disability on Channel Ten's official *Biggest Loser* forum could be thought of as a collective intelligence (Williams, 2009, p. 8) about the process of televisual identification. Online audiences in their exchanges bring in the reality of Selena's disability and how that impacts on her life – on and off the television programme. At the same time, online audiences point to the editing, framing practices and casting tropes of programmes like *The Biggest Loser,* and, as a consequence, they highlight how audiences are offered certain versions of the reality of life with a hearing impairment and obesity.

Our earlier discussion of the responses to Susan Boyle's performance revealed the ways in which audiences' investments in participants (and also characters) fluctuates. In their study of Somali–British young people's identity, Valentine and Sporton (2009, p. 736) point to the 'multiple, shifting and sometimes contradictory ways that individuals both identify and disidentify with other groups'. Likewise we found that online audiences feel an affinity for some contestants and an aversion to others, and like Valentine and Sporton's (p. 736) participants, online viewers feelings shift because of the ebb and flow of their 'emotional investment in different subject positions'.

The processes of identification and disidentification – reflected in the online comments we discussed throughout this chapter – are not binary opposites. They are linked in a dynamic nature of differences that are never fixed or complete, but change, crisscross, overlap and intersect (Medina, 2003, p. 659). de Swaan (1997, p. 106) explains that the process of identifying and disidentifying 'occupy two sides of an emotional triangle' – the base is made up of 'ignorance and indifference' because the 'vast majority of human beings are completely unknown to one another' (Butler, 2004, pp. 145–146). Similarly, media characters and participants are unknown to most audiences. None of us can know every single person in our entire community, so television provides an insight into people we do not know.

Conclusion

This chapter was concerned with audience activity, particularly identification and online activity. We concur with Sonia Livingstone (2004, p. 4), that the argument 'for the active television audience has probably been taken as far as it can go' and that theorization must branch out to consider other aspects such as the act of identifying and online activity. As Cohen's (2001, 2006) research reveals, identification is an internal process related to the viewer's experience of the television programme and their personal context. Although Cohen does not refer specifically to online audiences, his observations are a useful starting point to understanding the way online audiences engage with highly mediated characters.

Whereas the media typically essentializes disability, obesity and old age, attempting to reify these identity categories as facts rather than as culturally variable representations, online audiences shed light on how ordinary viewers identify and/or disidentify with characters possessing these traits. Examples of identifications cited include Susan Boyle in *Britain's Got Talent*, *The Biggest Loser* contestants Margie and Selena, and the so-called grumpy old men. Taking a cross-genre approach, this chapter explored the way audience members demonstrate their propensity to both identify and disidentify with characterisations of disability, obesity and ageing. Audiences will typically identify with a character when they consider they are similar or would like to be similar to that character – when audiences consider the character is not like them, or is like them in ways they don't want to be, they disidentify.

The following chapter draws on critical disability studies to argue that representations of disability draw on tacit knowledge to work as a narrative prosthesis (Mitchell & Snyder, 2000) on television and in online forums. The chapter critically examines narratives of disability in the series *Packed to the Rafters* and audience response to them on official forums and disability specific blogs. The discussion investigates the way online audiences negotiate and ask interpretive questions about what could be described as disabling televisual imagery.

PART II
Identifications

Chapter 5
Disability Drama

> We have been brought up with images of the village idiot, the pitiable invalid, the circus freak, the insane murderer, the disfigured outcast, the crippled villain. We have been raised to see people with disabilities as disgusting, repulsive, frightening, and even evil. We have been socialised to see people with disabilities as either impossible to love or desire, or the object of 'deviant' fetish (Lauredhel, 2009).

Images of disability feature in every television genre from news and current affairs to reality television and drama. Like Lauredhel, the blogger quoted above, audience members with disability recognize the limited ways they are represented on television – usually as criminals or outcasts – and the ways these images contribute to their social marginalization (Ross, 1997, p. 669). Recent analysis of disability on television has incorporated a consideration of audience response, as articulated on internet forums, to uncover the way audiences negotiate televisual images of disability according to their backgrounds and context (see Quinlan & Bates, 2008).

In this chapter we aim to further examine the way online audiences negotiate what could be described as disabling televisual imagery by examining representations of disability on the critically acclaimed Australian television drama *Packed to the Rafters*, along with online audience response to the portrayal. Audiences have overflowed the broadcast television boundaries of *Packed to the Rafters* – and indeed overflowed the overflow – to discuss the programme on sites beyond the official offerings. Whereas the series has provided thoughtful and provocative commentary on a number of social issues throughout its five seasons, in this chapter we focus in particular on Season 2.

We begin this chapter with an overview of the theorizing about the ways disability has been represented on television and popular media in order to situate this study within the current discourse of television and disability studies. The last major theorization of disability and television occurred in 1988 (Cumberbatch & Negrine, 1992) and focused on content analysis. Since this study, television has entered a post-broadcast era and undergone radical changes including tele-participation (Ross, 2009) and television overflow (Gray, 2008). Gray's notion of overflow has prompted discussion about the inclusion of people with disability. Quinlan and Bates (2008, p. 64) suggest blogging and forum participation captures both 'empowering and disempowering potentialities' for disability on television. Their analysis of blogger discourse about Heather Mills' appearance on *Dancing with the Stars* contends that disabling social values embedded in the text are absorbed by the audience. However, as the following discussion of audience response to *Packed to the Rafters* demonstrates, this is not always the case. The online discussions that predominately question the accuracy of *Packed to the Rafters'* depiction of cerebral palsy provide the opportunity to reflect on Gray's (2008) contention that television frames reality. We consider whether his conclusion that programmes either marginalize minority groups by replacing reality with fiction or invite audiences to 'seek out reality' (Gray, p. 121) can also be applied to *Packed to the Rafters*.

The second section of this chapter develops and explores these observations further through a critical analysis of disability tropes appearing on *Packed to the Rafters*. We provide a close reading of the development of the character Alex, a young man with cerebral palsy, who first entered the show as a minor character but then received major storylines in later episodes. In addition to this textual analysis, we will consider the discourses of disability that appear in online discussion of *Packed to the Rafters*. Because the show resonates with a female audience (Ward, O'Regan, & Goldsmith, 2010), we have selected for analysis discussion that appears on mothering forums, the disability blogosphere, particularly 'special needs' mothering blogs, and official Channel 7 forums. Two key themes have emerged in the online discourse:

- discussion about whether an actor with cerebral palsy should have been given the role
- debates over realism and the portrayal of cerebral palsy.

The narrative use of disability in television drama is crucial to the genre's functioning and audience interpretation of it. As Snyder and Mitchell (2010, p. 183) explain, 'the melodrama uses pathos towards bodily loss as the primary tool to evoke intense grief or sadness'. Thus disability has been used throughout all five seasons of *Packed to the Rafters* to evoke an emotional response of grief, sadness and the impression of domestic realism. Storylines have included anxiety, multiple sclerosis, HIV, Down's syndrome, cerebral palsy, epilepsy, depression and obsessive compulsive disorder. Therefore, within the drama–comedy genre in which *Packed to the Rafters* resides, disability offers a useful narrative tool to evoke an emotional response in the audience.

Disability on Television

Today's televisual images of disability mostly operate within paradigms of personal tragedy, punishment or miraculous cure. Whereas they represent a possible improvement to the 1990s tendency to use disability to terminate characters (Shakespeare, 1997), ultimately, these narratives exclude disability. These three narrative tropes were used in the first season of the Australian drama *Winners & Losers* (2011) through the character Doug. Doug, initially the convenient lover of commitment shy Sophie, experienced a personal tragedy – paralysis following a car accident with Sophie's friend Bec. The onset of his disability could be interpreted within the text as a punishment because the accident occurred the moment he began pursuing Bec, who had recently become single and was on the rebound, just as Sophie wanted to pursue an exclusive relationship with him. Finally, to complete the trope, Doug's disability was miraculously cured with, it would seem, minimal work. As an aside, Doug recuperated at Bec's house which had stairs leading to the front door – the question of how he navigated these stairs while using a wheelchair for mobility was never addressed.

Likewise, Carlos Solis's miraculous cure from blindness in Season 6 of *Desperate Housewives*, and Artie's dreams of walking in *Glee*, also reveal that, despite a general trend in wider society towards greater inclusion of people with disability, within the specific province of television, the problem is still portrayed as located in the damaged body. Within these popular television shows, disability is used as a narrative prosthesis (Mitchell & Snyder, 2000) to convey information about other characters.

Narrative Prosthesis: Packed to the Rafters and Televisual Social Issues

Disability is a representational identity and a 'prevalent characteristic of narrative discourses' (Mitchell & Snyder, 2000, p. 1). Narrative prosthesis refers to both the representation of disability itself and the meanings ascribed to it (p. 4). Mitchell and Snyder highlight the historical importance of disability to artistic portrayal since the sixteenth century and seek to expose the narrative use of disability to denote deviance and inferiority for example. *Packed to the Rafters* both uses disability as a narrative shorthand and provides space for characters with disabilities to make a connection with the audience who engage with these ideas, and each other, online. By assisting each other make meaning of the initial television text, online audiences influence the process of identification and contribute to television overflow.

Ranking as Australia's number one drama in its debut year, *Packed to the Rafters* is a consistent ratings winner. The show centres on would-be empty nesters Dave and Julie Rafter on the eve of their 25th wedding anniversary. Excited to be getting the house to themselves after their middle son Ben finally moves out (albeit only next door), Dave and Julie plan a romantic evening. However, their plans are thrown into chaos when their other children return home. The youngest, Nathan, and his wife Sammy move in to save money, while oldest, Rachel, returns to escape her abusive addict boyfriend. Julie's recently widowed father Ted also moves into the four bedroom one bathroom house following a series of panic attacks. This intergenerational household supporting one another in difficult economic and social circumstances resonated with Australian audiences during the global financial crisis (Ward et al., 2010).

Packed to the Rafters represents a key moment in Australian television drama production. It continues the ethos of domestic realism pioneered by internationally popular soaps, including *Neighbours* and *Home and Away*, by combining high production values with good writing to deliver a drama that captures the minutiae, messiness and ordinariness of domestic Australian life (Ward et al., 2010). It attempts to deal with themes and issues relevant to contemporary Australian life and the weekly one hour time slot gives the writers time to develop characterization and storyline. *Packed to the Rafters* has dealt with a number of social issues such as adoption, extra marital affairs, domestic violence, drug addiction, abortion and HIV diagnosis. Thoman (1987) argues that television most often covers social issues within the personal realm:

> Personal-social problems are primarily person-centered, that is, they consist of extraordinary circumstances that affect individuals or individual units of society – usually, crises in relationships or health. Every year the list gets longer but includes rape, spouse abuse, missing children, teen suicide, anorexia, cancer, AIDS, drug and alcohol addiction, mental illness, etc.

Many narratives on *Packed to the Rafters* deal with relationships and health, and disability has been frequently used as a representational identity and tool. To borrow Mitchell and Snyder's (2000, p. 1) words, disability serves as a 'character-making trope, a social category of deviance, a symbolic vehicle for meaning-making and cultural critique, and as an option in the narrative negotiation of disabled subjectivity' in *Packed to the Rafters*. The following analysis of *Packed to the Rafters* explores the representation and discussion of disability under these categories.

Although all of the main characters in *Packed to the Rafters* are white and non-disabled, disability permeates the programme and is central to several subplots and character arcs. We come to know what the family is like by the way they react to, and interact with, disability. Throughout *Packed to the Rafters*, disability works as a representational crutch – a symbolic vehicle for meaning making. This chapter focuses on the burgeoning relationship between Dave and Julie's daughter, Rachel Rafter, and Jake, an electrician who works for Dave at the family business Rafters Electrical. Alex, Jake's brother, who has cerebral palsy, is a symbolic vehicle for meaning making.

Packed to the Rafters has dealt with several social issues and the popularity of the series throughout Australia has led to a significant debate online regarding its educative potential. Online audiences both identify and disidentify with the social identities presented in the show. Identification with Alex himself is extremely rare – possibly because he is actually only a narrative prosthesis to convey information about the other characters such as Rachel and Jake. Yet, the Alex character introduced many people to cerebral palsy and encouraged audiences to seek out reality regarding this condition. To some extent this took place on the official Channel 7 forum (Bastow, 2009), but arguably was amplified on blog sites, when people with more experience with disability began to question and critique the construction of disability in the show.

Packed to the Rafters' casual introduction of difficult topics was described by one viewer as 'always authentic' (InTheWild, 2010), whereas another posited that the show often considered 'as many different opinions […] as possible' when tackling social issues such as 'abortion, DS, CP, HIV, unexpected pregnancy, MS' that other dramas wouldn't dare to represent (Anonymous, 2009). Often referred to as 'dramedy', *Packed to the Rafters* was described by Racer25 on *MediaSpy* (2009) as 'a great mix of comedic moments […] and more serious issues (Alex's cerebral palsy, Julie's middle-age pregnancy medical concerns, Chel's HIV-positive reveal)'. A consistent criticism of *Packed to the Rafters*, however, was the decision to cast a non-disabled actor in the role of disabled Alex.

Crip Drag

Disability bloggers, particularly those active on the *FWD for a Way Forward* blog, have written extensively about a phenomenon they describe as 'crip drag'. Crip drag refers to a non-disabled actor portraying a character with disability on television such as Artie from *Glee* and Alex from *Packed to the Rafters*. Blogger s.e. smith below argues that when television producers attempt to use disability to make a social comment they need to be more realistic in their portrayal. Using the decision to cast non-disabled Kevin McHale as disabled Artie Abrams on *Glee* as a case study, s.e. smith argues:

> I am angry about Artie and about the crip drag because there's no reason not to use a disabled actor; there are disabled actors who do meet the specs for that role. And I am grumpy because of the claims being made about the show; if Glee wants to congratulate itself for making social commentary, than it actually needs to make that commentary. One really good way to do that would have been to cast a disabled actor in that role. It is the discourse and framing which surround Glee which concern me (2010).

s.e. smith takes issue with *Glee* in particular because the show claims to offer a cultural critique. For example, accessibility is highlighted as an issue in 'Wheels', an episode that purports to centre on Artie. Until this episode,

Artie, who uses a wheelchair, did not feature in the narrative much beyond the occasional one liner. Then in 'Wheels', when the club can't afford to rent a wheelchair accessible bus to take the students to a singing competition, the non-disabled students are apathetic as to Artie's exclusion, suggesting he ask his father to drive him separately.

However, their teacher and mentor Will Schuster is adamant that the bus ride is a team building exercise that will prepare them for the competition. Artie, as a member of that team, must be included. As a consciousness raising exercise, Will forces the non-disabled members of the club to spend three hours a day in wheelchairs he purchased second hand from a nearby nursing home. Although 'Wheels' addresses problems regarding accessibility, it does so through non-disabled characters who struggle with access during their mandatory wheelchair time. For example, with all of his students using wheelchairs, Will discovers there is only one wheelchair accessible entrance to the school – on the far side of campus. After being alerted to this accessibility issue, Principal Figgins insists Sue Sylvester, Glee club nemesis and superstar cheerleading coach, hold open auditions for the cheerleading squad and, to Will's amazement, she invites Becky, a student with Down's syndrome, to join the squad. Down's syndrome and wheelchair use thus become conflated under the umbrella of accessibility issues in this episode of *Glee*.

Inspired by their experiences in wheelchairs, the Glee club decide to do a wheelchair number. Whereas this episode was embraced as a *sensitive* portrayal of disability by mainstream media and bloggers, cultural commentators active in the disability blogosphere slammed it as exploitative and tokenistic:

> There were so many problems with the way this episode handled disability that it's almost impossible to know where to start […] We got 'disability is inspiring', 'disability is a burden', 'appropriation of disability for a Very Special Learning Experience', 'faking disability', and 'see my sister has a disability so I'm not a bigot'. Here's the thing about tokenization, which is what this episode specialized in: It does nothing to advance the cause of people who live in marginalized bodies (s.e.smith, 2009).

s.e. smith's critique offers a good example of the way the disability movement disidentifies with the representation of disability on *Glee*. According to s.e. smith, *Glee* has been criticized since the beginning for using a non-disabled actor to portray Artie. The issue of actors without disability portraying disabled characters has been identified as a significant issue, but some online audiences who identify with disability have called for more nuance in the debate:

> I don't have an issue with an actor playing a character with a disability that the actor does not share. But, I do have an issue with disabled actors being so rarely

> cast. If disabled actors were regularly cast, just like any other actor, in a variety of roles, I don't think it would be a big deal if a disabled character were played by a non-disabled actor on occasion. Sadly, that's not the case. Inexcusable, really (LeeLee, 2009).

> Casting a disabled person to play a disabled person works if the person cast is the best actor for the job. So, […] if an actor with cerebral palsy was cast as a character where a disability was not either specified or important to the role then to me that would be the actor overcoming their disability and displaying their talent … i want to see an actor with a disability being a character in a story for the sake of the story because they are a great actor, now that would be good to see (Glenn, 2011).

s.e. smith argues that shows that claim to make a social comment on the inclusion of people with disability – for example, *Glee* should be held to the same standard of their own critique. *Packed to the Rafters* attempts to make this social critique on several occasions. For example, in Season 2 when pregnant Julie is undergoing prenatal screening for Down's syndrome on her unborn baby, the threat of disability is used as reason for termination. However, social aspects are brought into consciousness, such as when Dave suggests he is more worried about how society will treat a child with Down's syndrome, than he is about the prospect of having such a child. His admission that when growing up he felt like he didn't fit in, and that he is concerned that a child with Down's syndrome would be unloved, looked down on and rejected, could be read as critique of stigma. Yet, blood tests come back within the normal range and Dave and Julie decide not to undergo further testing. Again, disability works as a narrative prosthesis because the experience ultimately leads Dave to decide to search for his biological family. Whereas some viewers discussing this storyline tended to embrace the sentiment of the episode 'how lovely it would be to see littlies with DS in PTTR, for whatever reason' (jules363, 2009), others found the portrayal of disability tokenistic:

> I liked the whole debate about down syndrome children but I felt like I wasted my time watching that whole episode, yeah the acting was good and I'm sure it was all just to get [an award] for tackling such a topic but when they have an argument about it before even getting the tests back for then everything to be fine and wrapped up in a little bow it makes the audience feel stupid (pawlini, 2009).

The Down's syndrome episode 'Brave New World' was a particularly significant event in Season 2 of *Packed to the Rafters* for the community of self-described 'special needs mums' active on the *Thinking of Starting a Blog* site. Most agreed that they did not like the episode. Whereas Sarah (2009) commented that she was 'cross' watching it, Big Brother Little Sister (2009) claimed to 'scream at the screen' for the entire episode. Alison, the curator of *Thinking of Starting a Blog* (2009), wrote:

> I know for the writers it is just a story idea that they think will get ratings, but how does this affect people watching who have lived this? Especially the ones who didn't get the convenient TV ending of everything turning out fine? And why not have the story idea (shock, horror) that your child does have DS and you love them to bits and they are a delightful member of your family that you wouldn't swap for anything???

Thus the threat of Down's syndrome served as a character making trope offering a narrative prosthesis for Dave's reconnection with his biological mother. A similar prosthesis occurred as Rachel embarked on a new relationship with Jake.

Character Making Trope

Jake first mentions his 'cheeky brother' Alex in Episode 6 of Season 2 ('Little Arrows') when he and Rachel are accidently locked in a room together. Rumours circulated online that this brother would be disabled (*MediaSpy*, 2009). When Rachel and Jake finally embark on a serious relationship, Rachel becomes upset that she is not invited to Alex's birthday dinner (Episode 10, 'Ready to Catch You'). Jake explains to Rachel that birthdays are a special occasion for his brother Alex and their single mother Grace, and invites Rachel to their house for dinner the following night instead. When Alex meets Rachel at the front door, Rachel is visibly shocked. Alex says 'didn't Jake warn you I was CP?' Rachel, not knowing how to act or react, stammers 'cerebral palsy' and pretends that she knew. Alex and Jake are more jovial and make a play on the abbreviation of cerebral palsy – CP – to laugh that Alex is a 'cheeky prick'.

A scene inside the house is framed to show a number of trophies and football pictures in one corner of the shot, and, as conversation turns to Jake as a natural athlete, Alex mentions that he has the middle shelf for special swimming. Alex is different, he's not like Jake, and it appears that Grace is prouder of Jake than Alex. Conversations are difficult, even forced. When Alex tells Rachel he wants to be a presenter on a TV show, Rachel is encouraging towards this dream. However, Grace admonishes Rachel for not being honest. When Rachel, who works in advertising, protests that she's sure there are many examples of people with disabilities succeeding in the media industry, Grace challenges her to name one.

As mentioned above, Kristian Schmid, the actor portraying Alex, is not disabled. He describes his role as Alex as providing the impetus for a number of '"how am I going to deal with this?" subjects' (Knox, 2009a). Schmid also explains the reasons a disabled actor was not hired:

> I felt a bit of pressure, thinking it would be great if there was an actor who had cerebral palsy who could do it, but Australian television works so fast and there just wasn't anyone who had that experience. I was feeling slightly guilty about that, but people at The Spastic Centre said there was no way they could do more than a 12-hour day on set. Imagine having spasms all day long – which is a bit of a generalisation – and trying to concentrate on acting. After I've had a day on set playing Alex, my body is aching (2009).

Although pathways to employment and training opportunities for people with disabilities in Australian television are admittedly diverse, in reality there are still barriers arising from disabling attitudes and limited facilities that prevent people with disabilities from fully participating in this industry. Although some may have gained access to the industry because of their disability, they need to display talent above and beyond non-disabled people in order to maintain a career (Goggin & Newell, 2003). In addition people with disabilities may be passed over because producers believe that audiences will be attracted by big name actors, such as Schmid, who already have a following in the industry.

However, actors with cerebral palsy do exist. RJ Mitte, an actor on the American cult drama *Breaking Bad*, has cerebral palsy, like his character Walt Junior. Comments on the disability site *Ramp Up* applauded this authentic characterization over the use of crip drag that is found in *Packed to the Rafters*. This online audience was able to identify with the experiences of Mitte and Walt Junior:

> Look at RJ Mitte, who plays Walt Jr/Flynn on Breaking Bad; Mitte has mild cerebral palsy, as does Walt Jr, and that's about the end of it. His character arc involves much more than 'having cerebral palsy' – same, would you believe, as real live people living with disabilities! (Bastow, 2011).

The intention of the *Packed to the Rafters* scene in which Grace admonishes Rachel for falsely raising Alex's hopes of a career in television could be conceptualized as social criticism of the lack of inclusion of people with disability in the industry. However, if the producers were genuinely critical of the restriction of activity imposed on people who have impairments, then why not demonstrate that the prejudice is groundless by giving employment to an actor with cerebral palsy? At the time of Alex's first appearance, Australian television blogger Clem Bastow expressed disappointment that Alex was portrayed by a non-disabled actor:

> Kristian Schmid appeared on *Packed To The Rafters* […] in the episode Ready To Catch You […], playing 'hot tradie' Jake's 'cheeky' brother Alex. So far so run-of-the-mill for Seven's flagship dramedy, except for one notable difference: Alex has cerebral palsy. Kristian Schmid, it needn't be added, does not. The *Packed To The Rafters* messageboard […] lit up […] with debate about whether Schmid – and the show's writers – had done a good job or not; was it an accurate representation; should they have done it at all; what *is* cerebral palsy? While watching the episode […], I was plagued by one thought: why isn't an actor with cerebral palsy playing Alex? (2009).

Schmid, who admitted that his being cast in the role could be viewed as problematic, described his approach to the character:

> Look, it's interesting because normally you're just focused on the acting and hitting the right emotional keys, but when you're playing someone with any sort of disability or physical trait there's something else to think about. After talking to people with CP, it's about muscle spasms that you don't have a lot of control over. I'm generalising, but usually they have to concentrate extremely hard to control any twitches. There are so many things going on you get a similar look of concentration (cited in Santer, 2009).

As we argued in Chapter 2, people with disability have long been subjected to ridicule and are often a source of humour on television. Alex provides many moments of comic relief throughout *Packed to the Rafters*. Again, this feature of his characterisation was interpreted as both empowering and disempowering by online audiences.

Disability Humour

Beth Haller (2010) explains the importance of humour in television shows that feature characters with disability. As we discussed in Chapter 2, disability as a source of humour is an archetype of cultural representation. People with disability have been ridiculed through freak shows and stereotypes which focus on the body and its limitations. Haller notes that whereas once disability humour was destructive, it now has the potential to expose the diversity of people with disability. She argues that disability humour has moved through several stages and that following the work of disabled cartoonist John Callahan (*Quads!*, *Pelswick*) in the 1990s and 2000s people with disability took control of their own image. As a result, disability humour entered a new phase whereby society's disabling barriers are laughed at rather than people's individual limitations. This has had a flow-on affect on shows made by non-disabled television producers, allowing characters with disability to be treated in comedic fashion just like any other character. Haller claims that the current phase of disability humour builds 'bridges of understanding' between the disabled and non-disabled because 'everyone can laugh at our shared humour experiences, and having a disability is depicted as just another feature about human beings' (2010, p. 171). Haller draws on a number of television comedies and disabled comics to illustrate the way humour defies stereotypes to challenge preconceived notions about how people with disability should behave.

In *Packed to the Rafters* Alex often jokes about cerebral palsy, which makes Rachel very uncomfortable. Although some identified with the disability humour in *Packed to the Rafters*, others did not, expressing concern that Alex was being laughed at:

> I love how Kristin plays Alex my son is cerebral palsy and the jokes about themselves is spot on I actually thought the actor had C.P until my husband told me who he was. So good job Kristian (robyndaustin, 2009).

> the actor that portrays [Alex] annoys the hell out of me; the way he overacts it is horrible; its very forced; they should've recruited someone with an actual disability in my opinion rather than an actor who does a pretty poor job of playing someone with a disability; it feels like it is making a mockery of it (ryaneco, 2010).

Writing on the authorized site of the official Channel 7 *Packed to the Rafters* forum, robyndaustin applauds the realistic representation of a person with cerebral palsy, whereas ryaneco's post on *MediaSpy* posits that any representation presented by an actor who is not disabled must immediately invite ridicule.

In *Art and Lies?* Shakespeare (1999, p. 165) suggests an inherent danger with this kind of interpretation is that continual criticism or so-called 'disability correctness' will discourage people from representing disability at all:

> … while it is appropriate to critique simplistic and one-dimensional representations of disability, it is too easy to reject complex and nuanced works … which do not comply with politically charged notions of 'positive imagery'. There is a dangerous willingness to take offence at supposed violations of equality principles. Moreover, the desire for a positive representation can obscure the elements of cliché and distortion … which are heralded as 'good' portrayals.

The classification of positive and negative portrayals of disability is increasingly criticized within critical disability studies as being context specific and reductive (Ellis, 2008; Mitchell & Snyder, 2000) – as Shakespeare recommends, a more nuanced analysis takes into account production, text and reception. Our focus on online audiences attempts to analyse this nuance, as it allows consideration of both the way these characters are shaped (or not) as identification targets, and whether or not people identify with these characters' lives and experiences. This analysis enables a robust discussion of how disability is represented.

Token Character with Disability

Whereas Jake reassures Rachel that she just needs to be herself, the next time they see each other Grace tells Rachel that she knows her 'type' and doesn't like her. Grace continues her tirade against Rachel with the claim that Jake will always need to be there for Alex and Rachel would never be able to cope. Thus, Alex remains peripheral as the two women argue over the next few episodes. Forum audiences on the *MediaSpy* site tended towards sentimentality:

> I feel like he does a brilliant job portraying Alex. His character has been more than the token 'disabled guy' and that's been brilliant to see (Racer25, 2009).

Television is often criticized online for offering token representations of people with disability. For example, characters are criticized for not being integrated into the story world and not doing much to advance the narrative. *Glee* is frequently accused of offering tokenistic representations of disability. When this occurs, online audiences fail to identify with the character with a disability or they identify with weak sentiment.

Disability does not feature as a major storyline in the *Glee* episode entitled 'Laryngitis'. Instead, disability is used to make Rachel, a non-disabled character, feel better about her current predicament. When she faces losing her voice during a bout of tonsillitis, Finn, another non-disabled character takes her to see his friend Sean to offer some insight on how bad other people have it. Sean, who was injured in a game of gridiron football, is now quadriplegic. Throughout the episode Sean is always depicted semi-clothed and lying in bed. Sean tells Rachel that he misses his life, body and girls. As they talk, the camera takes in the *mise en scène* of Sean's impaired body and the paraphernalia of disability around the room, including his wheelchair and medication on the table. Rachel's identity crisis and fears, that her boyfriend Jessie won't love her if she becomes a 'vocal cripple', seem insignificant compared to Sean's suicide attempts and battles with insurance companies.

Although Sean is portrayed by Zack Weinstein, an actor with a disability, the place of Sean's character – solely as a means of reassuring the normality of a non-disabled star character – remains problematic. Furthermore, the fact that Rachel does not lose her voice renders Sean's lesson – that each person is more than the one thing they're good at in high school – somewhat moot.

This characterization sees the 'threat' of disability introduced and contained (Longmore, 2003; Richardson, 2010).

Sean's disability puts things into perspective for Rachel, a characterization that did not sit comfortably with media blogger Owen:

> I'm still uneasy about how Glee chooses to involve disabled characters, too. I'm sure it's well-meaning and it's certainly commendable, but they're always used as manipulative shorthand and moralizing. Here, Finn gets so annoyed by Rachel's grumbling about her throat infection that he takes her to see an old friend of his, a young man who was paralyzed below the chest after a tragic football accident. It was a kind of uncomfortable way to make Rachel count her blessings. She's fretting about losing her voice, this guy's lost his body – see? Do you see? It was all very blunt and a bit unnecessary. Plus, not for the first time, when Glee decides to have a scene where the disabled character sings, the show just can't resist segwaying into a better, more upbeat version of that song performed by its able-bodied cast -- somewhat undermining the point of letting a disabled character make a connection to the audience (2010).

The use of both non-disabled actors (Kevin McHale – Artie) and actors who have disability (Zack Weinstein – Sean; Lauren Potter – Becky) on *Glee* has been criticized for reinforcing problematic images of disability. In terms of narrative, characters are either peripheral, being used to support the main able bodied characters, or they dream of being non-disabled themselves.

Disabled Subjectivity

Discussion about Alex emerged on the Channel 7 *Packed to the Rafters* forum as well as on several dedicated cerebral palsy and disability specific blog sites. *Thinking of Starting a Blog* described the introduction of Alex as 'dangerous':

> There is a new character in the show – Jake (Rachel's boyfriend) whose brother has Cerebral Palsy – which is fine – good actually for people with disabilities to be portrayed on screen. However the character isn't played by an actor with CP, but someone pretending to have CP. VERY hard to do that tactfully if you ask me ... surely there are actual actors with CP out there that could have been used? The worst part of the storyline is that this character's mother is quite bitter and twisted. She comes across as very protective of her children, but in an aggressive, nasty way. Surely the media doesn't think that all us [Special Needs] mums are bitter and twisted from taking care of our children and worrying about their futures? Why not portray her as a loving, caring mum just like the main character of the show? (2009).

While this mother of a child with disability disidentifies with Grace, she identifies with Julie, apparently perceiving herself to be more like the loving, caring matriarch of the show. This disidentification with Grace's characterization was evident on a number of 'Special Needs' mothering forums. Blogger Terrible Palsy (cited below), also a parent of a child with cerebral palsy, expressed disappointment with the producer's decision to cast a non-disabled actor in the role of Alex. She describes being 'very confused' about whether *Packed to the Rafters* was her favourite television show anymore:

> What I love about the episode was the glass of white wine in Alex's hand as the family sat in the lounge room. Did anyone notice? What I don't like, is the actor's interpretation of a person who has cerebral palsy (2009).

These two bloggers, both mothers of children with disability, recognize the potentially positive impact of portraying cerebral palsy on-screen, for example in the comedic storylines afforded to Alex. However, there is disquiet about the extent of authenticity, or, more accurately, the lack thereof. They do not see Schmid as being able to accurately portray a person with cerebral palsy, and they do not see Grace's character as accurately portraying 'Special Needs Mums', that is, themselves. If the portrayal is not accurate, does the television representation merely move the community's view of people with disability from one false understanding to a new, but still arguably false, understanding?

Imcka28 posted a similar comment on the *Packed to the Rafters* official forum:

> I was completely unimpressed with how Packed to the Rafters introduced Jakes brother who has cerebral palsy. They had clearly not done their research into CP, as he was very very poorly represented. I work with people who have CP, and they are nothing like that. Quite an embarrassment to the disability community (2009).

This comment is a complex example of disidentification because Imcka was offended on behalf of the disability community, by virtue of professional association. The programme, however, encouraged people to seek out the reality of cerebral palsy. Through the process of meaning making about a television show and its overflow, the forum community was learning about the realities of life with cerebral palsy. Some bloggers issued a challenge to Imcka28 to explain how Alex should have been represented (kaz38178, 2009), while others expressed genuine interest in gaining perspective on a condition they knew nothing about (turtleslittle, 2009).

Alex garnered much discussion in the official forum, in particular regarding whether Schmid's portrayal was accurate, and what cerebral palsy was. Identification with disability played a significant role in people's interpretation. With the exclusion of Imcka28, the community members were mostly impressed by the authenticity of Alex's characterization, as these indicative comments illustrate:

> I am also touched by someone with CP on a daily basis and was very heartened by the way the producers and writers treated the character of Alex. I found him warm and funny and real. A great effort by everyone involved. The thing is about CP its very hard to compare cases as no two people are the same or have it to the same extent (lambertjessica, 2009).

> I thought Kristian Schmid was excellent in Packed to the Rafters. The way he played Alex was very realistic (janknowles, 2009).

> I have to agree, I thought Kristian was fantastic, a great actor. I actually cried he was so good, and I love Alex, he needs to be a main character and part of the family so we see more of him!! (wleesa, 2009).

Whereas several posters admitted to thinking the actor had cerebral palsy, others questioned whether cerebral palsy should have been represented at all and requested insight from people with some experience with the condition. The forum provided an opportunity for viewers of *Packed to the Rafters* to garner more information on what cerebral palsy was and possibly clear up some misinformation:

> The guy who played Alex [. . .] was heaps good. Hey sorry just a stupid question but what is cerebral palsy? I thought it was a brain condition (cerebral). Wouldn't that mean he had brain damage? And therefore wouldn't be able to talk properly? (turtleslittle, 2009).

> [I] was wondering about what exactly CP is and how it can affect people differently . . . any information is much appreciated ☺ (pttrfan01, 2009).

However, representation does not present a mirror image of the real world. Television is a signifying practice that relies on codes and conventions – realism is a construction. Although responses tended to proceed from a medicalized understanding of disability, the characterization got people talking and thinking about disability:

> From my understanding it depends on how badly the brain is affected by CP as to the condition of the person. Some people live full 'normal' lives if their condition is mild (Pandora878, 2009).

Pandora878 recommended forum members get in touch with another community member simple.blossom, who identified as having cerebral palsy. She offered this explanation:

> Cp is just a condition that is caused by brain damage normally when they [are] still in the mothers tummy, there are different degrees of cp depending on the amount of damage there is Hemiplegia, Diplegia and Quadriplegia. I have right sided Hemiplegia which affects my right hand and right leg – hav weakness – doesn't work the same as my left side. But I only hav a mild cp (2009).

Simple Blossom was able to provide a very simple explanation of cerebral palsy, allowing people to learn about disability while enjoying a television show. As Gray (2008) argues, analysis of what people do with the unreal allows us to understand the real. In earlier episodes, Alex works as a textual feature of meaning making as Rachel struggles to trust again while maintaining her fierce independence in the early stages of her relationship with Jake. Yet online audiences used this narrative prosthesis to interrogate the realities of cerebral palsy.

Progressively, Alex's characterization changes and he takes on a more leading role when Jake is diagnosed with epilepsy. In Episode 22 ('Nativity Play') of Season 2, Jake has a seizure when Alex is in New Zealand bungee jumping. Although totally absent from the narrative, Alex is significantly pursuing a more independent life at exactly the moment Jake is experiencing dependency for the first time. This is further explored thematically the following season when the tables are turned as Alex, supported and cared for by Jake all of his life, must provide support to Jake as he struggles with his own medical condition and the impact it has on his identity. Alex also offers Rachel a shoulder to cry on. This was celebrated on the *Walking is Overrated* blog:

> My personal opinion is they have done a very good job of developing this character in a not too schmaltzy manner. Issues around him maturing and gaining more independence, his feeling of loneliness and envy as all around him seem to be happily hooked up, and him now having to take some responsibility in respect to his older brother dealing with epilepsy … . (Rosemary, 2011).

As Rosemary indicates, Alex's characterization developed over the course of several seasons – to the point where he is also offered romantic interactions of his own. Thus Alex becomes a rounded character, and audiences move in and out of identifying with him according to their own experiences.

Conclusion

Television increasingly involves a two way communication using new media. However, as Turner cautions, it is reductive to view these online spaces as 'unproblematically empowering' (Turner, 2009, p. 147). Quinlan and Bates argue audience blogging and forum participation capture both 'empowering and disempowering potentialities' (2008, p. 64) with respect to disability on television. Their analysis of blogger discourse about Heather Mills appearance on *Dancing with the Stars* revealed the way representations of disabling social values are negotiated – sometimes accepted, sometimes rejected.

The emergence of empowering online communities, bonded by similar interests, can be seen in the blogging activity relating to *Packed to the Rafters*. *Packed to the Rafters* considers many issues relevant to domestic life, and as such has acquired followers on mothering forums as well as the official Channel 7 companion website. Discussion of key themes has also emerged in the Australian disability blogosphere. These internet texts demonstrate the importance of social identity and identification in the way audiences decode television texts.

In the next chapter we continue the discussion of the limited repertoires presented on television and responded to in new media, taking obesity as our case study. Larger bodies are increasingly visible on television yet differing messages are offered. Whereas some programmes, such as *The Biggest Loser*, claim that that thinner people are happier and freer than obese people, in *Mike & Molly* the message is that personal happiness is not a by-product of one's body size. In a media environment where increasingly ordinary bodies do not measure up, we are interested in what online audiences do with these conflicting messages.

Chapter 6
Obesity Makeover: Rejecting the Obese Body

> Contestants on The Biggest Loser are always going on and on about how they have 'gotten their life back' by losing weight, and I kind of get what they mean. Spending your life safely on your sofa can be a really compelling idea when the alternative means always being uncomfortable or unsure, encountering messages at every turn that your body is wrong or invalid, or worse, dealing with outright discrimination and vitriol because of your size. So yeah, one way to deal with that is to hide in your house and wait for the day that your body looks like everyone else's. Or you could just choose to live now (CarrieP, 2010).

During the last ten years there has been a gradual increase in on-air television programmes focusing on large body size. These programmes – *The Biggest Loser, Fat Camp, Dance Your Ass Off, Embarrassing Fat Bodies, Fat Actress* and *Extreme Makeover: Weight Loss Edition* – draw on a long history of verbal and visual markers to encourage both audience identification and disidentification. Most of these signifiers are excessive and reproduce socially disabling attitudes, such as the view that fat people are morally decrepit and out of control. Intriguingly, however, another crop of popular programmes have emerged such as *Mike & Molly, The King of Queens, The Practice* and *Gilmore Girls*, which embrace characters who just happen to be fat in leading roles. Yet, despite their claim to inclusion, many of the latter continue to draw on the standard verbal and visual markers – for example, there is a constant stream of fat jokes on *Mike & Molly*.

This chapter examines the way online audiences negotiate with what could be described as disabling televisual imagery in programmes such as *The Biggest Loser: Couples, Embarrassing Fat Bodies* and *Mike & Molly*. We draw from one official television site (Channel Ten, *The Biggest Loser* forum), one unofficial viewer-generated site (*Television Without Pity*) and one social movement site (*Big Fat Blog*) to consider the way online audiences respond to recent depictions of the obese body on *The Biggest Loser*. Contributors to these sites – both official and unofficial forums – have also discussed how obese bodies have been subjected to disabling imagery. This online discussion brings to light how televisual images offer a marketplace of ideas that can be publicly debated (Lorié, 2011, p. 36).

This chapter's main focus is the Australian Season 4 of *The Biggest Loser – The Biggest Loser: Couples* (2009) – and its companion website. One of the main claims made explicit in the programme – through the views of personal trainers and contestants – is that thinner people are *happier* and *freer* than obese people. In short, having a slim body is a pre-requisite to achieving personal happiness and freedom. This claim to happiness and freedom, however, is in direct opposition to what the contestants are required to internalize and impose on themselves to acquire that slim body.

We begin the chapter with a brief synopsis and background information about *The Biggest Loser* (2009). We follow this with a discussion about the recent trend in which the fat body is signified as the obese body. The representation of large body size or 'fat' characters has a long history of being signified as a 'mark of shame' and 'a stain' (Farrell, 2011, p. 26). Many of the verbal and visual signifiers used in earlier media, and discussed in Chapter 2, are circulated and re-purposed in twenty-first century televisual media. Television programmes rarely have a fat character in the lead role – usually fat characters operate in secondary roles to support the main character who is often much thinner. Alternatively, fat people are 'marvelled' at (Lloyd, 2010) in programmes such as *The Biggest Loser, Embarrassing Fat Bodies* and *Fat and Fatter*. Fat bodies are frequently subject to disciplining regimes in order to attain the ideal body.

The next section of the chapter moves to consider the televisual construction that thin people are freer and happier than obese people in the context of the socially disabling messages produced and reproduced on *The Biggest Loser: Couples* on air text. This idea becomes part of personal training discourse – a notion we also consider in this section. Foucault's work on disciplinary practices reveals how personal training discourse is used in makeover style programmes such as *The Biggest Loser*. Foucault's approach is useful to illuminate the techniques used by the trainers to discipline bodies in an attempt to attain the ideal body. One of those techniques is to transform contestant's personhood so they reject the obese body. For Murray (2005b, p. 155) a programme like *The Biggest Loser* confers personhood on the 'fat body', provided the person is engaging in a 'continual process of transformation, of becoming and, indeed, *un*becoming'. Ultimately, personhood is attained when the obese body is rejected.

The chapter then turns to examine the contestants and the online audience's comments about the weight loss journey on *The Biggest Loser* programme. Both contestants and forum participants see losing weight as paramount to increasing self-empowerment and self-love. Forum participants pinpoint the entertainment value of the programme, yet they also negotiate or resist the preferred message. We analyse the comments participants on the official *Biggest Loser* forum and contestants on the programme make about striving to attain the ideal body – and therefore consistently rejecting the obese body. Ultimately, the personal trainers and the contestants' phrases and statements are set in motion by programme makers to support the programme's claim that thinner people are *happier* and *freer* than obese people. The (re)production of disabling attitudes such as these reveal the limits of televisual (self) representation of the obese body.

The Biggest Loser: Background Information

The 2009 Australian series of *The Biggest Loser* format focuses on couples. The series consists of a host Ajay Rochester, two main trainers, Michelle Bridges and Shannan Ponton, and two additional trainers, Steve Willis (The Commando) and Emma Hutton (Emazon). The programme ratings increased after seven weeks; however, mainly on the Sunday night weigh-in episode and when the final winner was announced (OzTAM, 2009). These ratings are typical of reality television programmes that have a competition where contestants are eliminated.

The first episode in Season 4 was aired on Channel Ten on 1 February 2009 and the final episode on 27 April 2009. This particular series consisted of 75 episodes. Generally the weekly programme set-up comprised the following: Sunday episodes contained a major challenge conclusion, last chance training and weigh-in; Monday was elimination; Tuesday was 'warehouse' (teams choose between two food groups) or a challenge; Wednesday was 'temptation' (contestants are tempted with high calorie foods); Thursday was 'the walk' (contestants are given the power to change the game); and Friday was a major challenge. Essentially, these segments illustrate that the programme series is highly constructed, and they also demonstrate the programme's approach on how to challenge contestants to lose weight.

The Biggest Loser is also an excellent example of television overflow and the importance of tele-participation in the current era of television viewing. The official website is as important as the on air programme to the experience of *The Biggest Loser* as a source of entertainment. Online audiences use the website for a number of reasons such as motivating one another on their weight loss journey and critiquing the participants' behaviour and attitudes on the show. *The Biggest Loser* has also elicited response from the fat acceptance movement on the *Big Fat Blog*. As we discuss throughout this chapter, the tele-participation from official forum members is radically opposed to the online activists' views.

Undoubtedly, part of the programme's construction is to select contestants that a broad range of viewers can identify with. For instance, online audiences are likely to both identify and disidentify with each of the 10 couples who make up a total of 20 contestants at the start of the series. The competing couples include:

- The Mother and Daughter, Julie and Meaghan
- The Sisters, Holly and Melanie
- The Team Mates, Sean and Ben
- The Best Friends, Jeda and Jodi

- The Husband and Wife, Amanda and Stewart
- The Father and Daughter, Cameron and Samantha
- The In-Laws, Bob and Tiffany
- The Brothers, Andrew and Nathan
- The Newlyweds, Ramses and Tania, and
- The Work Mates, Sharif and Teresa (*The Biggest Loser*, 2009).

In addition, the contestants' ages range from 18 years (Melanie) to 56 years (Bob, the winner of the series). The catchphrase of the programme, is that if just one contestant can lose weight – with physical perseverance and the right mental attitude – everyone in Australia can, no matter how old they are! So the programme attempts to catch the attention of as many viewers as possible.

The contestants' class also functions as part of the production of makeover programmes like *The Biggest Loser*. Class is evident in that contestants who are selected to be on the programme are often from lower-middle-class backgrounds. Several studies show that makeover television promises advancement for lower-middle-class citizens (Fraser, 2007, pp. 188–189; Miller, 2008, p. 589; Redden, 2007, p. 155; Skeggs & Wood, 2008, p. 561) by suggesting that contestants have the power to transform themselves (Bratich, 2007, p. 17; Ouellette & Hay, 2008, pp. 471–472; Lewis, 2008, p. 443; Sender & Sullivan, 2008, p. 581). Even though the programme does not feature class as a major issue, the programme takes advantage of the aspirations of lower-middle-class contestants because nearly all the contestants are from working or lower-middle-class backgrounds.

Most contestants have white collar jobs in non-professional occupations where they sit down for most of their workday – for example, accounts manager (Holly), disability support officer (Nathan) and roadhouse owner (Bob). Similarly, when *The Biggest Loser* started in 2004 on American NBC, the contestants were also mainly from lower-middle-class backgrounds (Sender & Sullivan, 2008, p. 575).

When *The Biggest Loser* first aired in 2004, it was one of the first programmes to consider the experiences of obese people. Since then, obesity has become the topic of several television shows, traversing a wide range of genres.

Recent Television Depictions of the Obese Body

For example, as Elser and Stephenson (2011) note the topic of obesity was the theme of several different genres – namely docudramas, situation comedies, documentaries, and makeover reality programmes. Programme titles include *Mike & Molly, Huge, I Used to be fat, Heavy, More to Love, Supersize vs Superskinny, X-Weighted, The Last 10 Pounds, Big Medicine, Ruby, Shedding for the Wedding, Village on a Diet, Too fat for 15, Celebrity fit Club* (Elser & Stephenson). Like most of these programmes, *The Biggest Loser* constructs obese characters and participants as 'lacking in will power' (Farrell, 2011, p. 34). *The Biggest Loser* also perpetuates the view that obese people are undisciplined, sloppy and 'less likely to do productive work' (Greenberg, Eastin, Hofschire, Lachlan, & Brownell, 2003). Thus, in all of the programmes listed above the 'fat body' is seen as the 'uncivilized body' that lacks the self-control of the thin body (Richardson, 2010, p. 80). In *The Biggest Loser*, these characteristics are framed by the personal trainers and forum participants as lacking 'mental toughness'. Some contestants are depicted as giving in too easily when training becomes painful and temptation irresistible – such contestants are considered mentally weak and viewed as lacking self-awareness (*The Biggest Loser*, 2009). In our analysis of the programme, the trainers implicitly reinforce the stereotypical idea that the obese body is unhealthy, lazy, unproductive and unsuccessful.

Participants in programmes such as *The Biggest Loser* and *Fat and Fatter* are seen as 'letting themselves go' – of becoming a 'fat slob' (Brandon & Pritchard, 2011, p. 80; Richardson, 2010, p. 81). By Episode 6 of *The Biggest Loser: Couples* some of the contestants were constructed as indulgent, lazy and as giving in too easily. Views such as these can be traced back to early weight loss advocates (Farrell, 2011, p. 36); however, above all, associating 'fat' bodies with being unhealthy emerges in the late twentieth century (Brandon & Pritchard, p. 85; Farrell, p. 34; Heyes, 2007, p. 68). As Heyes (p. 68) points out, in health discourse and in popular culture discourse the assumption is 'that weight itself is a stand-in for health'. In other words, if a person who is overweight loses the weight this outcome solves their health problems. This belief is perpetuated on makeover programmes like *The Biggest Loser*. For example, one trainer, Michelle, equates slimness with health when she declares that the four top male contestants are moving 'into a future full of health and happiness' (Episode 53).

Contestants in *The Biggest Loser* are also visually constructed as abhorrent and disgusting (LeBesco cited in Brandon & Pritchard, 2011, p. 80) – this image is evident in the language used when contestants are confronted with big banner images of themselves to remind them of what they used to look like. For example, Holly's revulsion towards the larger than life images of her and her sister's former bodies is evident, as she comments: 'I never want to go back to those two big heifers' (Episode 13). All of the contestants react in a manner that reinforces stereotypical portrayals of obese bodies. And Shannan, one of the personal trainers, referred to his team as 'the sad people that walked into the show four weeks ago' (Episode 31).

Most of the contestants on *The Biggest Loser* are depicted as ordinary nice people, a typical televisual construction of fat people. Yet the same contestants are also portrayed as grotesque in different scenes throughout the series. This depiction occurs when contestants wear their Biggest Loser boot camp uniforms, and in the flashbacks of them in their underwear and consuming food. Images such as these can be used by producers to humiliate contestants on national and international television. Researchers and forum participants interpret this humiliation in two ways – one as a dubious representational strategy used to exploit the contestants' 'self-loathing' (Sender & Sullivan, 2008, pp. 577–579), the other as a key motivational and transformational step (DietVader, 2009b; workingout, 2009).

Indeed, the role humiliation plays in weight loss transformation is a question discussed in several threads on the website forum, but never clearly resolved. One line of thinking is that no amount of money would be worth the indignity of revealing the over-weight body on national television in its underwear:

> I don't know … nothing would motivate me to appear on national tv wearing only my bra and undies and then go wibbly-wobbling through weeks of physical torture until I'd slimmed down enough to have half my skin removed as it was flapping around in the breeze and frightening children. **shudders dramatically** (inarastarte, 2009).

> Why do the cruel producers make the contestants strip for weigh-ins. I'll tell you why … so viewers can be judgemental when they expose their huge butts, cottage cheese cellulite, overhanging guts and man boobs. I've watched TBL with others and all I ever hear is 'OH MY GOD'. I'm sure most of the contestants would prefer to cover up to hide their imperfections. So why not allow them to keep a bit of dignity in front of a national TV audience (TheDanaCrew, 2009).

These forum posts recognize the links between current representations of the obese body and the earlier examples of obesity as spectacle in the freak show. However, another line of thinking is that the act of appearing semi-naked on national television signals the depth of an individual's commitment to the weight loss challenge. As such, it is a key motivational and transformational step, especially in the case of the first weigh-in:

> Yeah i can see ur point i wouldn't fancy standing on national tv in my bra or knickers either!!! **But** i honestly think as hard as that would be and as hard as the first weigh in would be its all part of losing weight. I struggle with my weight but no one knows how much i weigh not even my partner, nor my mother!!! So standing like that in front of australia would be a massive motivation for me to prove to everyone i will change. it would be a massive wake up call. I would love to audition for the show! (workingout, 2009).

Exploiting contestants' own self-loathing was seen by some as unwarranted. Many people on *The Biggest Loser* forum – and in other media – state that it was not necessary to humiliate contestants at weigh-in and during the commando's army style training with the clothes they wore. The crop-top sports bra and aerobic shorts that the women wear accentuate their rolls of flesh and skin. The men take their t-shirts off to weigh-in right up to the final episodes (Episode 67), thereby revealing excessive rolls of flesh and male breasts. It is not clear why it was necessary for contestants to wear tight and minimum clothing when they weigh-in, especially clothing that is not flattering. At other times there are flashback segments (usually in black and white) of contestants in their underwear at home looking in a mirror at their body. The camera always focuses on rolls of flesh. Continually showing this – even after contestants have lost significant weight – further accentuates their humiliation. This disabling televisual imagery endorses demeaning depictions of large size people, and audiences do absorb such socially disabling attitudes about large size bodies. However, not all online audiences were of the same mind about the televisual imagery, which reveals that representations of disabling social values are negotiated – sometimes taken on board, sometimes rejected.

Interestingly, UK participants on the programme *Embarrassing Fat Bodies* show their genitals, breasts, stomach and nude bodies on national as well as international television – showing much more than contestants on *The Biggest Loser.* When they begin interacting with the doctors on the programme, participants on *Embarrassing Fat Bodies* immediately become patients – their body parts are probed and inspected both by the medical doctor and the television camera. Thus their bodies are under both the televisual and medical gaze. For instance, Lisa who is about 114 kg – 'twice the weight she should be' – comes to the mobile clinic to see Dr Pixie McKenna (Episode 3, Season 1). Lisa and Dr Pixie sit facing each other; however, it is Dr Pixie who directs the interview and asks the probing questions. The doctor measures the patient and provides the expert information about vital statistics, bio-age and treatment. During the interview, Lisa answers Dr Pixie's questions timidly and briefly. When the doctor is inspecting and measuring Lisa's weight, the camera zooms in and shows parts of her body. Now a patient, Lisa barely speaks throughout this segment. Similarly, when Dr Dawn Harper medically examines Yolanda (the patient), the camera focuses on her body parts; however, Dr Harper's face is in the shot when she is speaking (Episode 3, Season 1). Ultimately, however, the televisual gaze dominates, as these indicative scenes demonstrate. Presumably this representation of the exposed fat body is for viewers' entertainment.

It is interesting to compare the foregoing with images of an obese body in *Mike & Molly* outside the reality genre. After analyzing Season 1, we noted that Mike and Molly have the largest body size and are the main characters, they are portrayed as normal people who depict real experiences (see *Television Without Pity* forum participants' comments), and viewers are positioned to identify with Mike and Molly (most forum participants identified with Molly then Mike). For instance snowbunny54 on the *Television Without Pity* forum expressed the sentiments of several other posters:

> Dear Writers, you have made significant progress so far. Please continue. I guess it should have been expected that the writers would treat (us) fat folks as easy fodder for the joke machine. I can see now that you are maturing in your storyline and character development. I am glad that you have discovered that we have feelings, desires, jobs, sex, etc., just like other sized people (2010).

Yet as one forum poster on *Television Without Pity* notes producers of *Mike & Molly* depict the fat body differently to *The Biggest Loser* as well as slim bodies on television. MrsLovett1979 comments:

> I generally liked the episode, there were MUCH fewer fat jokes. However, it did display a huge double-standard when it comes to fat people on TV. When Mike and Molly were in his bed, having just had sex, Molly was wearing a freaking long-sleeved shirt! Normally, in a scene like that, the woman would be in lingerie, or sometimes even just a bra (the show does air at 9:30), but never, ever a long-sleeved shirt. Who puts a long-sleeved shirt on right after sex? Or wears it during? I think TPTB are afraid to have her show any skin, because 'OMG, a fat body is so ugly!' The Biggest Loser has been showing fat men and women without their shirts on for years, I guess it's ok when you're beating them into acceptable size, but not when it's a sign of a fat person's sexuality. BTW, Mike was in a t-shirt, which still covers most of his body, but at least isn't long-sleeved (2010).

Thus, the depiction of the two main characters reveals it is possible to put forward different representations of obese characters, yet, the representation of Mike and Molly in the bedroom is dissimilar to that of slim bodies. Compared to *The Biggest Loser* contestants, however, Mike and Molly appear happier and freer from loneliness because their relationship develops (as opposed to feeling freer because they are losing weight).

Samantha Murray, a key writer in the fat acceptance movement, claims that in much of the discussion about the construction of the 'fat body', the overriding view in Western narratives marks this as 'a site of moral decay and failure' (2005a, p. 111). As Murray points out, the fat body is 'hypervisible in terms of its mass in relation to the thinner bodies that surround it' (2005b, p. 157). Since individual and societal reaction to large body size is a widespread response to 'visible difference', Murray says, one expects disgust and cruel retorts 'to "fat" bodies' inside and beyond the medical clinic (2007, pp. 363, 371). Murray highlights that people's reactions to fat bodies draws on their 'tacit body knowledges', which is partly produced through medical discourse, media representations and societal attitudes (p. 370). Even contestants on *The Biggest Loser* make self-disparaging comments about their large-sized bodies. One of the contestants, Jodi, shares her daughter's fear that Jodi was 'growing into a monster', and Jodi responds 'I am' (Episode 75). Jodi reveals in her response that she expects others to find her body disgusting, and, as a consequence, Jodi does not consider herself a person, at least not until she begins her weight loss journey.

The Biggest Loser: Thinner People are Happier and Freer than Obese People

Televisual media frequently essentializes characters' and/or participants' identities – this is especially so for fat bodies. For example, in shows such as *The Biggest Loser* and *Embarrassing Fat Bodies,* fat bodies are constantly measured using scientific devices in an attempt to prove what is obese. Rarely do programmes such as these consider how medical science partly informs the cultural construction of obese bodies. Forum participants of *The Biggest Loser: Couples* (2009), for instance, complained that the contestants were not really obese – for this online audience, the bodies were not 'big' enough (see the thread 'Too Light to be Contestants', 2009). Similarly, fat acceptance movement participants, commenting on the US, production, said that 'some of the participants aren't even particularly fat' (QitelRemel, 2004, see the thread 'NBC's The Biggest Loser').

Most comments by personal trainers, contestants and official forum participants suggest that the fat, obese body needs to be remade, because it is less desirable, less productive, less healthy and less worthy, in other words, less morally acceptable, than the slimmer body (see also Sender & Sullivan, 2008, pp. 580–581). Likewise television tends to reinforce the idea that the slim body reflects a life that is whole, future orientated and under control. One of the main claims the programme makes – through the pronouncements of personal trainers and the contestants – is that thinner people are *happier* and *freer* than obese people. Often being fat is likened to being in a prison. (It was the younger contestants who talked in this way; the contestants who were over 50 – Julie, Cameron and Bob – rarely spoke like this). In this view, contestants and forum participants identify with messages in the programme.

Frequently in *The Biggest Loser* the view of the personal trainers and the contestants is that thinner people are freer. This view is socially disabling because freedom is defined in a very narrow sense. Freedom is dependent only on one's body size according to *The Biggest Loser* discourse. Being freer has a specific meaning within the programme – thinner people are freer to go to the beach, live the lifestyle they choose, go out in public without being judged because of their weight (Meaghan, Episode 59), and be active with their children (Andrew, Episode 19). This freedom does not take into account the disabling impact of other people's prejudice. Early on in the series Meaghan says 'once I am free from my own emotions, nothing will stop me' (Episode 7). Later she goes on to say that she has 'never felt free' because she has always been overweight (Episode 59). Meaghan proclaims that she would 'literally shut' her bedroom door and would not come out because she felt so judged about her weight (Episode 59). Tiffany, after successfully completing the super challenge to create new memories, says 'I feel free' (Episode 57) because 'I have conquered my fears' (Episode 59). Towards the end of the series, Sharif discloses that he thought he was 'disgusting' and that he did not realize 'how unhappy' he was, but now he knows what 'it means to be free' (Episode 69). Yet for Sharif being free means 'you don't have self-loathing, you have self-respect' (Episode 69). In a later episode, when contestants are having a total body makeover, Sharif remarks that he and his wife will 'have a life other people are envious of' – losing weight for him meant that his life would 'be perfect' (Episode 51). In another episode Shannan says to Sharif: 'You're the man who has been hidden away from life by fat' (Episode 74). Michelle adds: '[Sharif] is now the man he always wanted to be and he truly is free' (Episode 74).

Yet this claim to freedom does not account for the new regulations contestants must internalize and impose on themselves – do intense exercise after consuming excess calories, weigh their food, calculate the fat/carbohydrate/protein/calorie content of every morsel of food they place in their mouth. Thus, through internalizing the training and discipline, the individual is able to be regimented – and as a consequence feel *free* – because they no longer have to ponder choices. In a nutshell, they must internalize the correct course of action (Foucault, 2005, p. 357) in order to maintain their slim body both inside *The Biggest Loser* camp and on the outside.

The contestants talk mainly about freedom in the psychological sense. Yet as their bodies diminish in size, they appear to replace one kind of mental prison for another. Ostensibly, the first prison for most of the contestants was emotional and psychological, one where they were imprisoned through their own self-beliefs and their desire for food. Once contestants slim down and become a thin body, their prison takes the form of obsessing about food and subjecting themselves to the surveillance of trainers, forum participants, and people in the public realm. Furthermore, contestants must regulate their bodies through intensive daily exercise in order to maintain their new slim selves and through physical and mental perseverance, to control their desire for food. Thus persevering to try and attain the ideal slim body requires mental as well as physical stamina. Surpassing and maintaining their weight loss goal is only possible if contestants internalize practices to regulate their mind and body, consume diet products, exercise equipment, gym membership etc., over a lifetime. When we consider what the contestants face in light of Foucault, attaining their weight loss goals becomes a lifelong project on the self (2005, p. 315) as well as 'the promise of a better future' (Fraser, 2007, p. 182). However, they aim for a body that is rarely attainable.

The other main message from the programme and the contestants themselves is that thin people are *happier*. For instance, Meaghan (Episode 7), speaking about her 6.3 kilo weight loss says, 'makes me a hell of a lot happier. The happier I get, the freer I will feel'. When Sean was evicted, his parting words were that he is a lot 'more confident', a 'thinner and happier' person (Episode 26). Tiffany (Episode 40), another contestant, says she wants to be like past winners – Alison, Cosi and Sam – who are happy because they are 'slim'. Tiffany comments that these contestants have 'got their life on track'. From these quotes, it can be argued that contestants have successfully identified with the messages in the programme and the personal trainers' mantras (discussed in the next section).

In the programme, reference is continually made to contestants being able to continue their weight loss journey at home. In this context, the 'weight loss journey' is seen as a lifelong commitment to the disciplinary practices of losing weight once an individual has the necessary skills and attitudes – the 'right equipment' (Foucault, 2005, p. 326). The major focus in the programme (often repeated by forum participants) is having 'mental toughness' – the ability to keep going despite bodily pain, urges and desires. Further sharing of information – about calories, exercise, body mass index (BMI), and weight loss practices via *The Biggest Loser* official forums – is important in acquiring skills and attitudes for the individual in the present and in the future. In short, contestants and forum participants seek to attain a body of knowledge that they can materially draw on immediately and as their journey progresses.

However, contestants may become *un-free* because of the financial outlay to transform themselves and stay slim. Transformation of the self involves expensive 'consumption' (Redden, 2008, p. 486). The weight loss industry is a multi-billon dollar business in Western societies. And merchandising on *The Biggest Loser* official website is a part of that billion dollar industry (see http://www.thebiggestloser.com.au/the-club.htm).

In addition, weight loss discourse encompasses purchasing weight loss products such as personal trainers, replacement meals (when one is too busy to cook), exercise equipment, gym membership, low fat cookbooks, and, at the extreme end, paying for fat-removal surgery (unless the programme or government health services covers the cost as in *Extreme Makeover: Weight Loss Edition* and *Embarrassing Fat Bodies*). Weight loss entails material costs in which the individual continually outlays money; however, the programme presents this lifelong project on the self as a simple matter of mental toughness.

Transforming the Obese Body Through Personal Training Discourse

Discussions throughout this book have shown how disabled, obese and old bodies are depicted as not measuring up to 'the standards of normality' (Wendell, 1996, p. 89). Like disabled and old bodies, the fat body in the televisual text is contrasted with an 'ideal' body type, which is conflated onto a 'physical' body (Wendell, p. 86). We argue that essential to television programming is maintaining the ideal thin body; however, most ideal bodies that appear on television are underweight compared to the general population (Fouts & Burggraf, 2000, p. 929; Fouts & Vaughan, 2002, p. 439). In this section we reveal that by transforming themselves, the contestants uphold this ideal. In programmes like *The Biggest Loser*, the contestants do this transforming through personal training discourse.

Contestants exemplify how personal training discourse works as they start achieving their goal of losing weight and getting fitter through exercise. In this way, personal training discourse is exemplified when the body is transformed materially through specific techniques (Foucault, 2005, p. 322). Techniques include memorizing calorie and fat content in food, vigorous fat burning exercise, personal mantras and affirmations. For instance, an often quoted mantra by the personal trainers on *The Biggest Loser* programme is that there is a 'slim' person inside the layers of flesh just waiting to get out of 'the prison of fat'. Contestants internalize this idea and repeat it at different times throughout the programme.

The makeover genre has specific ingredients, which enable contestants to make this self-transformation and internalize the personal training techniques. These ingredients include personal trainers as experts, family members' and contestants' reflexivity, the new self celebrated in photo shoots, contestants winning challenges, and motivational symbols such as the (slimmer) dream outfit. These ingredients are used as signs throughout the programme to reinforce the idea that the slim body is the standard to reach – these include the afore-mentioned contestants' dream outfit enclosed in a glass cabinet, the diminishing weight celebrated in photo shoots, and contestants' emotional response to cardboard cut-outs of their initial body size.

One particular tactic the programme employs is to use the personal trainers as mentors. For instance, in *The Biggest Loser* programme the personal trainers take the view that mental toughness and psychological strength will enable contestants to lose weight. So in order to achieve this, the contestants are frequently bombarded by trainers with the language and equipment the contestants need to develop this attitude. To begin with, contestants are exhorted to develop a relationship with themselves, and by doing so build up the 'equipment' to deal with their life – that is, the psychological strategies and physical fitness to achieve and sustain their weight loss (Foucault, 2005, p. 326). The relationship and equipment are essential for the individual to develop a life plan and carry it out, so that ultimately the self becomes the 'equipment'. The personal trainers (Michelle and Shannan) offer the contestants lessons through the repetition of phrases common in personal training and self-help discourse such as: 'no more excuses' (Michelle); 'show us what you're made of, dig deep' (Michelle); 'look it in the eye, stare it down and face it' (Michelle); 'time to take control of your life' (Shannan); 'have no regrets' (Shannan); 'embrace the philosophy' (Shannan); 'learn how to suck it up' (Shannan); and 'what we can do is control what we're doing' (Shannan).

These phrases are the personal trainers' 'lessons' – that is, 'phrases' that contestants and participants have 'really heard or read, really remembered, repeated, written and rewritten' (see Foucault's discussion of the athlete 2005, p. 323). The contestants use the phrases they have 'spoken' to motivate themselves (Foucault, p. 323), and to continue working on themselves in order to achieve the ideal. The ideal in personal training discourse is to 'surpass' one's self as well as to 'surpass' others, namely through weight loss and fitness levels. For instance, the winner of the 2009 series, Bob Herdsman, at the finale said that he and his daughter-in-law 'never set out to beat anybody', we 'just set out to conquer ourselves' (Episode 75). Tiffany (the runner up) commented, 'I was never against Bob, I was always against myself' (Episode 75). So, for contestants Bob and Tiffany, it was more important to surpass their own self, than to outstrip others. To achieve their goal, contestants and forum participants learn the language, so they can and do recite what the trainers say.

Through internalizing the trainers' phrases, so that they are 'ready to hand' (Foucault, 2005, p. 326), contestants and forum participants can routinely draw on them in any situation, at any time. As a consequence, the phrases are the equipment – the disciplinary practices of losing weight – in which contestants can transform themselves into thinner people. During the process, contestants begin rejecting their obese bodies. The discourses are embedded in the training techniques, so they become what Foucault refers to as 'a memory of activity' as well as 'a memory of action' for the contestants (p. 326). By being able to recall an activity or action, contestants can 'act' as they have been trained 'to act' by the trainers. The skills and knowledge the contestants gain from training becomes the armoury against gaining weight in their everyday lives (Foucault, p. 326).

However, only some contestants internalize the personal training phrases in their striving towards the ideal slim body. Even though most contestants put on weight after leaving *The Biggest Loser* programme (anecdotal evidence reveals this), it does not mean they have not internalized the discourse. Therefore, by continuing to identify with the ideal slim body, contestants can persistently spurn their obese body. As a consequence, the contestants on *The Biggest Loser* construct themselves as a lifelong 'project on the self' (McGee cited in Miller, 2008, p. 587). Hence, immediate weight loss is not essential to being successful.

Contestants are considered successful if they construct themselves as striving to be slim to increase their self respect, and/or their family's and the nation's. *The Biggest Loser* contestants mostly talk about transforming themselves for their families rather than for the nation. It is the case, however, that on occasion contestants sometimes make a call for other citizens to be 'like them' (Bob, Julie and Tiffany) – explicitly to identify with the contestants' project of weight loss –

and take up the challenge of caring more for themselves and their families. Bob and Julie often pointed out that, as people aged 50 plus, they are happy to be an 'inspiration'. This can be seen in Bob's comment, that if people think 'He's 56 years old. If he can do it, we can do it' (Episode 16). When Bob's wife joins the conversation on the official forum thread, 'TBL Weight Loss Record, Shannan Happy, Real Weight Loss Expert Unhappy' (2009), she reveals that Bob's weight loss had been unsuccessful so far. For her, Bob participating in this programme now means he 'has a chance at least' to learn 'about diet and exercise', and, at the same time, improve his health (Littlejlh, see the thread 'Saggy Skin', 2009a; 2009b). One forum participant, on the same thread, identifying with Bob's challenge to lose weight, responds that they are inspired by his huge weight loss and hard work (Gordita, 2009). Personal training discourse places emphasis on inspiring others to train, to lose weight and to get fit.

As intimated above, personal trainers consider the contestants have a moral duty to lose weight for their families and for the nation. Michelle, Shannan and presenter Ajay take a fervent view about the nation's problem with obesity. Throughout the series Michelle explains why it is important for contestants and viewers to lose weight as a pledge to the nation. Shannan refers to the contestant's duty to confess to the nation when he says: 'Time to stand in front of the nation and bear your soul' (Episode 1). In their appeals, the trainers urge viewers and contestants to disidentify with the obese body. Further, Ajay claims that Julie has 'proven to everyone here and everyone in Australia' that it is 'never too late to change' (Episode 68). In the finale episode, Ajay (Episode 75) says to Bob: 'and not only have you saved your own life, but by doing what you have done, you will no doubt save thousands and thousands of people's lives'.

Similarly, the doctor–presenters in *Embarrassing Fat Bodies* continually point to how much obese bodies cost the National Health Service (NHS in the UK) – insinuating that if obesity keeps going up the NHS will collapse. As a consequence, people who remain obese, are constructed as morally deficient because their (over)weight affects their families' health and the nation's health system (Jutel, 2005). Online audiences discuss these and other issues on *The Biggest Loser* official forum. Forum participants adopt the personal training discourse whereas fat acceptance bloggers reject it and espouse a different view. Ultimately however, identification and disidentification is dependent on online audiences' beliefs regarding empowerment and entertainment.

Online Audience Dis/Identification with Contestants: Self-empowerment and Entertainment

Both contestants and forum participants see losing weight as paramount to increasing self-empowerment. Contestants in *The Biggest Loser* often commented at the weekly weigh-ins how empowered they felt as their weight went down. For example, Cameron (Episode 7) could 'not believe the change' in his life; Nathan (Episode 43) felt 'every single day' he was 'earning a bit more of [his] life back'; Tiffany (Episode 43) felt 'strong' and 'empowered'; Cameron (Episode 61) commented that he will 'go home a different person'; Jodi (Episode 63) believed the programme gave her a 'kick start' and felt she could now do anything; and Bob remarked that 'everyday I am here I increase my life out there' (Episode 74). So, alongside transforming themselves for family, learning about how to maintain weight through exercise and dieting was seen by contestants and forum participants alike as a path to personal 'self-regulation and empowerment' (Ouellette & Hay, 2008, p. 476).

Furthermore, losing weight for many contestants is equated with 'learning to love themselves', which is another path to self-empowerment. An empowerment they could not achieve when their body was obese. For many contestants, loving themselves was equated with feeling proud of their achievements. For example, Amanda (Episode 17) remarks on feeling 'proud' of herself; Julie (Episode 28) comments she feels 'proud' of herself 'so far' (Episode 35); Tiffany (Episode 37) feels 'so proud' of her 'achievement'; Teresa (Episode 37) observes she is enjoying the 'pride' she has in herself 'now'; and Sean (Episode 52) began to feel 'very confident with the way' he was looking and no longer doubting himself.

Contestants on the programme as well as forum participants speak about continuing their weight loss journey at home as a lifetime commitment to loving themselves and their family. By attaining knowledge about nutrition, calories and exercise, and learning about one's eating habits, as well as consuming foods promoted as good choices in the advertisements and product placement (Redden, 2008, p. 486), the contestants (and the online audiences) can metamorphose themself (Bratich, 2007, p. 18) – in the case of *The Biggest Loser* from the ugly duckling to the swan. The never-ending project is a constant desire to attain an ideal slim body. Contestants, however, uphold the prevalent view that slimness is the cultural ideal in Western society. From this perspective, contestants affirm the moral divide (Foucault, 1977) between those who uphold the body ideal and those who do not, and, in doing so, they reinforce disabling attitudes about body size.

The idea that people can only love themselves if they have a slim body is not accepted by the fat acceptance movement. In stark contrast to the programme and the contestants' view, the online fat acceptance movement commit to loving their bodies – no matter what size – as outlined by the blogger DeeLeigh:

> Fat acceptance is not about trying to change your body. It's about taking joy in the body you already have. Fat acceptance isn't a rebellion against 'The Biggest Loser'. The movement has been around for forty years, and it's about social justice and about valuing human diversity. Fat acceptance is not about trying to

> be fat. It's about not hating our already fat bodies, and about fighting anti-fat stereotypes, prejudice and discrimination (2010).

Here DeeLeigh offers reasons why the fat acceptance movement disidentifies with nearly all representations of the fat body on television. This blogger takes the view that television programmes like *The Biggest Loser* attempt to persuade audiences to reject and hate the obese body. Another blogger in a thread 'Fat on Reality TV' contends that reality programmes like *The Biggest Loser* are loved by viewers – 'the public' – because of 'the amount of ridicule the shows can dish out' (Maria, 2004). And the 'ridicule' is 'all in the interest of entertainment' (paul, 2004).

Programmes like *The Biggest Loser* are geared more towards entertainment, since melodrama is a large part of the content, than towards providing factual information about how to lose weight and/or the health risks of gaining excessive weight (see Dovey, 2000, pp. 17, 97). Yet we found that most online viewers of television programmes such as *The Biggest Loser* are fairly aware of programme makers' techniques (see also Kavka, 2008; Skeggs & Wood, 2008). These online viewers are observant of how reality television programmes are highly edited, casting is an important element, contestants' personalities are constructed (DietVader, 2009a; 2009b) through the editing process, and that contestants' bodies are contrived as grotesque (see also Sender & Sullivan, 2008, p. 579). Many forum participants on the official *The Biggest Loser* website took a similar position. For instance, storm-boy pointed out: 'it's edited to the max, scenes cut and spliced between days and weeks – all to provide the entertainment factor' (2009); DietVader opined that it has to be 'dramatic enough to entertain the audience' (2009a); and Cactusfreek expressed the view that many of the challenges humiliate the contestants who are 'the spectacles' and 'it's horrible!' (2009). Two forum participants commented on why they watched *The Biggest Loser:*

> i watch purely for the entertainment value of human nature, how they behave, how they interact and their personalities to say they are going to do something and stick to it (as we all know how freakin hard that is!) (almitywife, 2009).

> So why do we watch it? Because us fatties want to emotionaly connect with these contestants in order to find the inspiration to do something about it ourselves (Cactusfreek, 2009).

These forum participants reveal a paradox central to the success of the makeover genre. Makeover programmes rely on viewers identifying with some contestants and disidentifying with others.

Most forum participants disidentified with Cameron because they found his attitude offensive. Cameron's attitude came to the fore in the 'Warehouse Challenge' (Episode 33) when the contestants cycle on a spin bike, earning 10 cents per kilometre to pay for their food. The contestants divide the task up, with each contestant responsible for two hours (in the 24 hours). Cameron initially refuses to participate in the challenge – his view is that 'If you don't exercise, you just don't need food'. However, his daughter Sammy feels embarrassed and frustrated by her father's attitude. When the trainers arrive to check-out how the contestants are going with the challenge, the camera zooms in on Cameron who is looking irate with his arms folded, and shaking his head – sitting on the couch some distance away from the other contestants. Most forum participants disidentified with Cameron and his point of view – nearly all empathized with Sammy (his daughter), for having to contend with her father's negative attitude. For instance, forum posters in the thread 'Suck it up Cam and Ride Yer Bike' (2009) called Cameron a sook, bratty, childish, spoilt, mentally soft, annoying, a master of evasion, and not a team player. In their remarks, participants implied that Cameron has the opposite qualities to Bob (the winner of the series). Thus, despite the knowledge that *The Biggest Loser* is heavily constructed, forum participants continue to embrace the preferred message in this instance.

Although *The Biggest Loser* programme aims to entertain, some viewers use the programme for more than entertainment. According to comments on the forum, some participants regard the programme as a motivation tool – doing their exercises while the programme is on, and eating after the programme, in order to lose weight. As forum participants testified: 'I never feel hungry after watching an episode, I always feel like I wanna get up and exercise' (jungle0005, 2009); 'I end up doing my abs and push ups during the program' (cathur, 2009). And one very motivated forum participant said:

> yes I am hungry but I am on the treadmill with BL is on and then I have my dinner. I find that BL motivates me. Every year I lose weight while the show is on and then go into Big Brother and put some of it back on because I do what the people do on BB and sit around eating … lol (domesticqueen, 2009).

Some online audience members on *The Biggest Loser* official forum discussed the weight loss practices used by the trainers in the programme, as well as what the forum participants considered were appropriate practices to discipline the obese body. Forum participants affirmed some of the trainers' techniques – for instance, some saw the Commando's approach as motivational because it was an accepted institutional approach (army), others disliked Michele's psychological approach. Overall, forum participants were more critical of the female trainer's techniques than those of her male counterpart.

Other forum participants admitted that watching the show made little difference to their eating and exercise regimes (brideofhorror, 2009; nickeroo, 2009; sub101, 2009). It is impossible to essentialize – some online audiences are not swayed by the melodrama and editing techniques, and do not identify with the programme contestants. Yet they participate online. This suggests that tele-participation (Ross, 2009) has become an integral part of the viewing experience.

Conclusion

The fat body is represented by many of the verbal and visual signifiers used in earlier media. These signs are circulated and repurposed in twenty-first century televisual media. The online audience in their comments about *The Biggest Loser* reveal how viewers can draw on tacit knowledge – in particular statements they hear in the televisual media and in the everyday – about fat people. Throughout this chapter we have explored the way fat bodies are commonly represented to shape the development of this tacit knowledge.

This chapter revealed how television production choices and signs, exemplified by *The Biggest Loser*, affect how contestants are discussed by viewers. We highlighted that essential to a makeover programme is the ability to transform and advance oneself. Drawing on Foucault's disciplinary practices, we pointed to the preponderance of personal training discourse to help contestants transform themselves. The lessons and phrases given to the contestants by the trainers are the equipment to continue a life-long quest of weight loss.

In our analysis of *The Biggest Loser*, we found that television tends to reinforce the idea that the slim body is indicative of a life that is healthy and has a future. One of the main claims the programme makes – through the personal trainers and the contestants – is that thinner people are *happier* and *freer* than obese people. However, this mantra does not take into account the regulations and restrictions contestants must adhere to remain slim.

In the next chapter we continue our discussion of the ideal body presented on television and responded to in new media, making ageing our focus. Despite the increased representation of older characters on television, idealized images of youthfulness persist and the makeover genre again promises an unattainable ideal body. In this context, we argue, the increasing visibility of older bodies on television – mainly the young–old – does open up discussion about the processes of ageing rather than continually focusing on old age as a fixed state. Yet, the socially disabling stereotypes about old age persist.

Chapter 7
Ageing Transformations: Embracing the 'Young–Old' Body

> I loved Grumpy Old Men – did not think it was sad just true – I think older people should speak up more about all the annoying things that go on. I'm tired of being interrupted by phone calls selling me something, automated answering when all you want is a human being, and clothes designed for under 23 yr olds. I could go on but fear I will be called a grumpy old woman. (I don't care) Bye (bonnie, 2005).

> Horrible bloody shows. Both are frighteningly positive arguments for mandatory euthanasia. They encourage a certain desire for stovepipe pants, mod haircuts & Mildara Hermitage. Anything to distance oneself from identification with such losers (earle qaeda ®, 2010a).

Depictions of ageing continue to be informed by stereotypical and essentialized discourses in most contemporary Western television programmes. Many older characters are in cameo roles – older characters that do appear often look youthful, healthy and active. For example, *Cougar Town*, *10 Years Younger in 10 Days* and *Absolutely Fabulous* typically focus on midlife characters, specifically the 'young–old' (Bradley & Longino, 2001, p. 17), who are about to face growing older. Rarely do the old–old appear in main roles, and the deep–old only appear as a signifier of a body in decline. The mainstream television examples we have selected for analysis throughout this chapter focus on middle-aged peoples' anxieties about growing older, rather than old people/characters per se.

Television typically tries to quantify age, alongside disability and obesity. However, it can be argued that continually trying to enumerate what *is* old ignores the way in which ageing is culturally moulded. How people think about ageing indicates their cultural standpoint. Nancy Signorielli (2004) draws attention to the significance of television as a medium for shaping social and personal perceptions of age and ageing. For her, television represents characters in all phases of their lives and, in terms of ageing, it imparts 'an almost inescapable set of messages' about what it means to be old (Signorielli, p. 280). We explore these messages throughout this chapter to argue images of ageing evoke negativity and fear. Whereas engagement with consumer culture is offered as a way to neutralize this fear, online responses show how audiences sometimes do not concur with the view of ageing presented on television. In spite of this, many audience members reinforce the view that the ageing body needs to be regulated and that makeover television could help people do this.

The chapter begins by exploring the question what is old age? As Fishman (2010) points out, what was identified as old in previous generations might be considered middle-aged now. Yet, the 'state of being old' is presented as a generalized idea in the televisual media and often depicted by an old body. This body is reviled because it signifies decrepitude, senility, decline and death (Woodward, 1991, pp.18-19) as reflected in popular representations of ageing such as *One Foot in the Grave*. Thus on television the old body is symbolically annihilated, and as a consequence oldness has less value than youthfulness and/or the youthful body.

The chapter then turns to a consideration of the discourse of 'positive aging' (Featherstone & Wernick, 1995, pp. 6, 10, 13) as it has influenced Western views about how individuals should physically age – namely that they ought to appear healthy, attractive and youthful. The so-called young–old has become the standard portrayal of older characters in contemporary television programmes. This is a depiction not based on chronological age, but on youthful looking characters who are physically as well as mentally active and healthy (Chivers, 2011). On television a youthful look (cf. Woodward) dominates because most producers assume the audience is young(er) than the ageing or old characters they represent. So even when the representations of elderly people do appear, their representations are constructed for an assumed younger audience. Television's focus on maintaining a youthful appearance disregards the socially and culturally disabling attitudes Western people generally hold about growing older and older people.

The chapter ends with a case study of the makeover programme *10 Years Younger in 10 Days*. Here, we examine the ways in which online audiences on the lifestyle website *Vogue* (and also *Whirlpool*) invest in and engage with social meanings of age. This programme's online audience also provides valuable insights about (dis)identifications with the process of ageing. We are particularly interested in this programme because of the way it constructs ageing as an undesirable outcome of living life, such as having children, grandchildren and physically demanding but rewarding jobs. Although the programme *10 Years Younger in 10 Days* encourages audiences to disidentify with the appearance of the old body, online audiences still detect that growing old is a gradual development rather than an end point of life. For example, the online audience recognize contestants' ageing process within their lifestyles, work and family, yet, the same audience supports the proposition that the older body should be made-over so it looks youthful.

Furthermore, according to online audiences, programmes of this genre have a role in advising viewers about their grooming, diet and clothing choices so they can look more youthful. Although online audiences criticize the television programme for including cosmetic procedures, they also maintain that everyone should make an effort to remain youthful looking, which supports the modern view that being young–old means not *letting yourself go*. Two social conundrums are revealed in the programme – acknowledging the ageing process and not letting yourself go. Here having to appear young–old – at all times – becomes an emotional and psychological prison. Like the contestants on *The Biggest Loser* (discussed in the previous chapter), the individual's desire to appear youthful takes the form of obsessing about grooming and body shape. Individuals also subject themselves to the surveillance of the televisual gaze and people in the public realm. Thus internalizing the young–old standard as well as the regimen to live up to the ideal youthful body becomes socially disabling for most people.

What is Old? Television Images of Youthfulness vs Oldness

Growing old is something most people expect to occur. Even so ageing is not the same experience for everybody as comments like those made by bonnie and earle qaeda at the opening of this chapter show. Unlike other identity markers such as race, gender, disability and obesity, according to Kathleen Woodward (1999, p. x) age is 'the one difference we are all likely to live into'. Yet a sense of fear surrounds the notion of growing older. Programmes like *10 Years Younger in 10 Days* tap into this fear about ageing. Whereas studies have shown that older people do not necessarily fear old age – for instance many older people report enjoying retirement, experiencing satisfaction and wellbeing in later life (Degges-White & Myers, 2006) – younger people tend to be less optimistic about the prospect of ageing (Revera Inc & International Federation on Ageing, 2012). Indeed media and popular culture have tended to portray ageing characters in negative ways. According to Cristofovici (1999) limited and negative portrayals of ageing diminish the ways in which ordinary people can imagine and engage with the process of ageing.

Western societies attempt to cope with anxieties about ageing by classifying oldness and youthfulness as 'polar opposites' (Woodward, 1991, p. 6). This thinking highly values youthfulness over oldness as a lived experience. *Hot in Cleveland* promotes this point of view. In this situation comedy, three LA women of a certain age are forced to make an emergency landing in Cleveland (en route to Paris). When they realize they are still considered *hot* in Cleveland, they decide to stay on. These characters are cast as the young–old because they embody the youthful–older person image – they are active, socially engaged, have slim, youthful bodies and wear in-vogue clothes. In each episode, the three main female characters are fashionably dressed in chic sun dresses, cami-tops, tight jeans and stylish accessories. Even though all the female actors are over

50 years of age, they are made-up to appear ten years younger – that is, to look as if they are 40-year-old single women. *Hot in Cleveland's* premise is that age is defined variously, depending on location, as evident in Joy's (one of the characters) quip: 'moving to Cleveland has extended our shelf life by 20 years' (Episode, 'Hot for Lawyer'). This programme supports the notion that ageing is a cultural construction, yet, it also maintains that youthfulness is the preferred model.

Woodward observes that when youth becomes the dominant term, two things occur. First, the term youthfulness becomes a viewpoint that is a 'moveable' sign within our psyche, second, old age becomes the fixed term or the end point that is seen as immovable (Woodward, 1991, p. 6). This opinion is shared by Cathrine Degnen (2007, p. 70) who agrees that people prefer to identify with youthfulness, which is seen as a malleable state – very few people self-identify as old. Our own research supports these findings. Many online audiences disidentify with old bodies, but not necessarily with individual older contestants or the process of growing older. This is explored in further detail below, using the programme *10 Years Younger in 10 Days* as a case study.

Television media attempts to essentialize and quantify old age, even though as Degnen (2007, p. 70) asserts, old age is a relational concept that cannot be defined just by physical appearance or chronological changes. A case that illustrates Degnen's point is the use of the term 'elderly' by television researchers. In his research, Bell (1992) categorized elderly as people on television older than 55, and actors in their 60s at the time the programmes were made. Yet Vernon et al. (1991, p. 59) regards '65 years of age' (and older) to be elderly. Featherstone and Wernick (1995, p. 13) talk about 'deep old age', which could be interpreted as 80 years plus. From observations, in 2013, people aged 55 and over (up to at least 75 years) do not call themselves elderly – either on television or in everyday life. Of course the term elderly has different meanings for different groups and contexts – for example, elderly characters on television are often depicted as no longer able to live independent lives. For instance, the BBC comedy series *Getting On* is set on a geriatric ward for over 80-year-old female patients in a London hospital. The series is written by Jo Brand, Joanna Scanlan and Vicki Pepperdine who also play the medical staff. The task of nursing their frail elderly patients is complicated by the demands of hospital bureaucracy and human resource management. (In this programme *getting on* also implies having to deal with the complexities of Britain's healthcare system).

The real action is the hospital employees' negotiation and management of the system, with the elderly and dying patients forming the backdrop. The camera frequently pans around the ward portraying the vacant expressions of frail elderly women (many have dementia), who appear bemused by the antics of the staff. For example, the opening scene of Series 1 focuses on the death of 87-year-old, Lily. Sister Flixter (Joanna Scanlan) holds Lily's hand as she passes away while at the same time checking and responding to her mobile phone messages. In the context of the show, Sister Flixter's multi-tasking appears realistic, and it presents life and death as just another administrative function.

Some of the online audience on *The British Comedy Guide* forums comment on the authenticity of the show's representation of hospital procedures and its treatment of distasteful and taboo content (Mark, 2010; Miss CTree, 2010; Wout Thielemans, 2011). These online participants identify with the setting. Yet others contest the programme's realistic portrayal of old age; ultimately, they contend that the representation is ageist. For example, chipolata (2010) describes *Getting On* as a 'bleak and nihilistic portrait of old age … The patients seem little more than ciphers, just there to stare into space, mess themselves or die'. Tim Walker (2010), another online participant, echoes this sentiment:

> Getting On … views illness and death in old age through a filter, saying that it must be pure bleakness, daily boredom and suffering. The patients in the show are rarely, if ever, given a chance to speak for themselves. It adopts a stereotypical 'youthful' view of old age and death, projecting the fears and values of younger generations onto old people. Plenty (the majority actually) of elderly patients go into hospital for whatever treatment, get compassionately treated, then leave again. That story doesn't fit the agenda of the show, but it happens all the time and this should at least be acknowledged by creators and reviewers. Yes, chronic illness and death in old age may be banal in one sense, but this show decides that an elderly person's final days on the planet are undignified and worthless. Not so. There is something ever-so-slightly ageist about this show which I don't like very much.

In a survey by the Pew Research in 2009, people were asked about their expectations versus reality of growing older in America. Unsurprisingly, different age groups had different perceptions of what constituted old age. Although it was generally agreed that old age began at about 70 (the average age was 68), respondents identified a variety of features that signified the beginnings of old age – 'failing health, an inability to live independently, an inability to drive, [and] difficulty with stairs' (Pew Research, 2009). Respondents pointed to how one's physical abilities are also affected by their environment. Wendell (1996, pp. 39–40) explains how people's environment structures their physical world, noting that:

> … poor architectural planning creates physical obstacles for people who use wheelchairs but also for people who can walk but cannot walk far or cannot climb stairs, for people who cannot open doors, and for people who can do all these things but only at the cost of pain or an expenditure of energy they can ill afford.

So what is old? As indicated above, a plethora of sub-categories of old age have been identified by various researchers – the young–old, the old–old, the disabled elderly, the very old, the frail elderly, and deep–old age which in itself demonstrates the contested boundary of old age (Degnen, 2007). Kessler, Rakoczy and Staudinger (2004) argue that categories such as the 'young–old' (people between 60–80 years of age) and the 'old–old' (people over 80 years of age) reflect the terms the third and fourth ages coined by social historian Richard Laslett (cited in Holstein, Parks, & Waymack, 2011, p. 67). Laslett equates the third age with the expanding period between the end of paid employment and the onset of declining health (cited in Holstein et al., p. 67). Holstein et al. (p. 67) take Laslett's earlier ideas further and assert that what was once referred to as 'old age' is now more aptly referred to as 'older ages'. Vesperi (1985, p. 24) takes a similar view to Degnen, arguing that old age is a cultural construct and researchers should consider the context of ageing rather than old age as a discrete category.

The Discourse of Positive Ageing

Recently the idea of positive ageing has emerged as a discourse that has influenced Western views about getting old. This influence has extended to televisual media. According to Hodgetts et al. (2003, p. 419), positive ageing has three key tenets – older people should live independent, physically active and socially active lives, and that particular values and beliefs form as a result of positive ageing discourse. For instance, one belief is that individuals are *allowed* to age on condition that they keep physically healthy, attractive and youthful. Another is that the individual is responsible for his or her ageing, that the ageing process is very 'self-determined' (Hodgetts et al., p. 419). Most televisual characters depicted as the active elderly – for example, Betty White's character Elka in *Hot in Cleveland* – exemplify this notion of '"successful" ageing' (Hodgetts et al., p. 419). Successful ageing in this context means internalizing the disabling belief system of positive ageing.

When older characters look significantly younger, they embody the tenets of positive ageing (Featherstone & Wernick, 1995). Positive ageing comes from gerontology studies and is a celebratory position that champions positive images of ageing and older people (Featherstone & Wernick). As Featherstone and Hepworth (1995) explain, the discourse of positive ageing counters the traditional view of linking ageing with 'illness, disability, disengagement and decline' and replaces that link with images of active, healthy, youthful older people (p. 31). Although this position celebrates the ageing process, it ignores how the discourse can be socially disabling for older people because it does not interrogate the social and structural process that gives rise to the negative images. The images of positive aging in the media, Featherstone and Wernick

(p. 11) note, have been taken up by a consumer culture that promotes techniques and products to repair the ageing body. These range from developing fitness regimes to paying for invasive cosmetic surgery. As a result, advertizing and product placement urge older people – both men and women – to look more youthful (p. 11). Yet these images 'do not eliminate ageist messages' (Wilkinson & Ferraro, 2004, p. 345) and they may in fact perpetuate ableist messages.

So, while the older person who flourishes is applauded for thriving and flourishing as they age, those who fail to be physically fit and socially active risk being rebuked, ridiculed or pitied for not meeting the standard (Hodgetts et al., 2003, p. 419; Holstein et al., 2011, p. 67). On television, there are many instances of older characters who are depicted as 'the inactive elderly' – for instance, people who are overweight, disabled, and sick – these are represented as a body that is in decline and dependent on others for care (Featherstone & Wernick, 1995; Gullette, 1997, p. 14; Hodgetts et al., 2003, p. 419). These older characters are considered to have failed to meet the criteria of positive ageing, and are often portrayed in nursing homes, or in bed at home. It is in these depictions that the positive ageing discourse becomes a socially disabling message.

On today's television, active and youthful older people or characters are the measure of normality. Our discussion of *Hot in Cleveland* (previous section) and *10 Years Younger in 10 Days* (in the next section) reveals the following elements that support the norm – the rise of a consumer culture (Bradley & Longino, 2001, p. 18), current research and advances in biomedical and cosmetic surgery. As Heyes notes, in the US women 'make up 82% of cosmetic surgery patients' (2007, p. 104). The norm of youthful looking women on television has been accompanied by the view that a woman's youthfulness is largely linked to appearance – that is, body shape, grooming, styling and make-up artistry. Likewise, we note that men who are ageing are also targets of a consumer culture focused on having a youthful appearance.

For example, in *10 Years Younger in 10 Days* ageing and appearing old are essentialized. For the programme makers and the public, old age can be visibly quantified. At the beginning of each episode, members of the public guess a couple's age based on their appearance. This age then becomes their 'actual age' for the duration of the episode (Coupland, 2009). Therefore, the programme is based on envisaging physical appearance as the prime indicator of biological age. This viewpoint constructs the older body to be spurned, and, in the process, accentuates the limitations of *seeing* age.

10 Years Younger in 10 Days: Seeing Ageing

10 Years Younger in 10 Days promotes the view that we (the audience) need to manage the visible ageing body and that looking physically old is undesirable.

Each episode features a couple whose physical age is transformed by industry specialists through a regime of exercise, diet, grooming and styling tips, as well as minor cosmetic procedures. Before and after their makeovers, the couples are put on public display so people on the street can guess their age. Style teams on the programme compete to make individual contestants appear ten years younger than the initial estimate given by members of the public. As the episodes develop, the contestants' anxieties are reduced about the initial public estimations of their age because of the experts' promises to help them reverse and transform their ageing bodies. Thus the programme promotes the young–old as the standard portrayal for any ageing bodies.

The 2009 Australian series of *10 Years Younger in 10 Days* is based on the British series. The series consists of a host Sonia Kruger, and ten experts who comprise of a Grooming Coach, Hair Stylist(s), Stylist(s), Beauty and Make-Up Artist, Plastic Surgeon, Cosmetic Dentist(s), and Personal Trainer. The programme rated in the top five in the first week (Knox, 2009b) and as it was scheduled in the 9.30 pm time slot it rated well. However, as the season progressed the ratings dropped. Despite high ratings for the series opening the Seven Network did not renew the series for a second season.

The first episode in Season 1 aired on the Seven Network on 21st April 2009 and the final episode on 30th June 2009. In each episode one husband and wife couple (mostly from rural Australia) are given the opportunity to reclaim and restore their confidence through an entire makeover. This particular series consisted of 11 episodes. Generally the weekly programme set-up comprised the following: the presentation of the makeover challenge; the individual contestant exhibited publicly in a glass case (before and after their makeovers); the separation of the couple into opponent teams; the style teams compete and work against the clock; the before and after photographs; and the final reveal of the participants' signature styles. The experts have ten days to achieve their goal of transforming each contestant to look 10 years younger. The team that comes closest wins the competition.

The show follows the makeover genre (Bratich, 2007, p. 17) in suggesting that contestants have the power to transform themselves. Transformation of the self often involves making choices that largely involve 'consumption' (Redden, 2008, p. 486), such as cosmetic surgery. The programme's viewpoint is that self-renewal is brought about by the transformation of the body. Indeed the view that looking ten years younger will improve self esteem and relationships is emphasized. Thus physical appearance is instrumental in goal achievement.

We choose to analyse the *Vogue* responses to *10 Years Younger in 10 Days* because this forum focuses on body image and fashion. This forum exemplifies Williams' (2009, p. 43) idea of a 'collective intelligence' in which an online community (even a temporary one) is able to 'pool their information and experiences in ways that create new knowledge available to the entire group'.

In their feedback about *10 Years Younger in 10 Days*, *Vogue* forum members contribute what they have learnt from watching other makeover programmes. In their discussion of the programme, online audiences negotiate the televisual depictions of ageing as they thrash out the degree to which any ageing body can be or should be transformed. Furthermore, the conversation on the forum illustrates how online audiences can move between a process of identifying and disidentifying.

Most *Vogue* forum participants accept that it is the individual's responsibility to keep themselves feeling and looking young. The emphasis here is on appearing visibly young. For online audiences, the media has a role to play to achieve this goal, by advising viewers on how to manage the ageing body and how to retain a youthful look for ageing bodies; however, this emphasis reinforces the belief that ageing is a state of decline (see Gullette, 1997).

Aged by Lifestyle, Work and Family

Whereas *10 Years Younger in 10 Days* implies that contestants on the programme have aged more than necessary because of ill-informed personal choices, their relationship to family and work also contributes to the ageing process. Most contestants are Anglo-Australians who work in non-professional occupations, such as the retail industry, trades and small business, and are selected because of their enduring heterosexual relationships. The programme suggests that contestants have aged because of their intense involvement in the social networks of everyday life. Yet, the programme fails to recognize that these are the very routines and bonds that contribute to a full and meaningful life and the target audience identifies with these aspects. Intriguingly these are the experiences that obese contestants on *The Biggest Loser: Singles* (discussed in Chapter 4) felt they miss out on – those contestants were in effect made-over so they could begin to participate in such social networks.

The Australian programme also focuses on the country and city divide. In the Australian collective imagination there is a schism between cities as centres of culture, style and consumerism (feminized spaces) (Fiske, Hodge, & Turner, 1987, p. 115; Lambert, 2010) – and rural areas as cultureless spaces, defined by adversity, hard work and mateship (Bryant & Pini, 2009). The programme *10 Years Younger in 10 Days* uses the iconic city landscape of Sydney to reinforce the otherness of its contestants. The contestants – by virtue of living in rural Australia and their unstylish appearance – are portrayed as different from those who belong in the city. The setting of the city is presented as a transformational space, which both accentuates the contestants' pre-makeover rural identities and allows for their youthful self to be reconfigured.

The presenter Sonia Kruger reinforces this divide in her quips (Episode 1) that the objective is to 'bring glamour back to the coal mines'. The audience learns, for example, that Annette – being a coalminer's wife from country Queensland – (Episode 1) occupies 'a man's world' where 'even the dog's a bloke' and that few opportunities exist for 'feminine' pursuits like shopping. Neil, her partner, is pictured operating heavy mining equipment and throughout the episode Neil is referred to as Hagrid and Ned Kelly.

Sonia Kruger points out to contestants that it is their lifestyle, or their job, or their role as a grandmother that has worn them out and made them old. And in Episode 2, Andrea and Wayne's biker lifestyle is presented as having contributed to their weathered appearance. Described as 'bikers from the bush', Andrea is characterized as a 'tomboy' who needs to reclaim her pre-baby shape. Then in Episode 3 the narrative for Donald and Julie is 'a life devoted to kids and grandkids' has 'left them stuck in a time warp'. John and Tracey (Episode 4) are 'childhood sweethearts whose social life is suffering'. Although John wears an eyebrow ring and socializes with his children, a makeover is deemed necessary to restore Tracey's self-confidence. Heavy work demands have contributed to the premature ageing of Kylie and Chris (Episode 5), and Natasha and Michael (Episode 6), whereas in the case of Juanita and John (Episode 9), 20 years of marriage has resulted in John 'letting himself go'. Described as 'the New South Wales Central Coast's answer to "the Brady Bunch"', Robyn and Michael (Episode 10) have been aged by the challenges of raising a large blended family.

In the programme, therefore, working-class, rural or regional contestants are more likely to be positioned as victims of the ageing process because of hard working lifestyles and lack of knowledge and resources about how to care for their ageing bodies. Online audiences noted this city (stylish) versus country (unstylish) stereotypes. However, even though they did not identify with the unstylish (old and scruffy) looking contestants, audiences did not accept contestants' lack of youthful image as a reason to belittle them. For this *Vogue* online audience, lifestyle and ageing should be made compatible – that is, seen within a context – rather than just adopting the latest style so a contestant looks more youthful. For example, several online participants spot the inappropriateness of the makeovers for contestants' lifestyles – for instance, comments were made that urban metrosexual chic is not suitable for a coalminer. This mismatch is noted by this online forum participant:

> The clothes that they put them in were SO unsuitable for where they live … I'm not saying that people in country towns cannot get dressed up but what they needed was to know how to dress nicely when they are casual and going out as a family (Adele04, 2009).

Online audiences in their response to the programme's class depictions reacted, but did not necessarily reflect on how ageing is affected by contestants' class. For example, one participant's viewpoint about the selection of contestants for the programme is that 'Its like they go walking through a trailer park to pick out which couple to style next for the show!' (Electrifried, 2009). Another posted that the show should be renamed, 'How to turn a Bogan into a Normal Person' (bartybates, 2009). For example, in her review for *The Age* newspaper, Catherine Deveny discloses how thoroughly dubious the show's fantasy of youthful reinvention is because it is based on a cynical assessment of class:

> Ten Years Younger In Ten Days should be called You're Old And Ugly. We're Not. 'We can make you look a little less ugly and old for a moment, with a mammoth effort and humiliation, then as soon as you get back to your tragic suburban homes, your diet of takeaways, fags and instant coffee, your tracky dacks and your jobs in pizza shops, mines and pet shops, you'll snap back to your former ugliness and you'll know, for sure, there is no happily ever after. You're ugly. And so's your family. Get over it […]' (2009).

In this reading, Deveny points to the ways the makeover journey capitalizes on the aspirations of working-class participants and, in doing so, the programme reproduces their disadvantage as television entertainment. Yet even though many of the online audience may disidentify with the contestants' class, they do, however, identify with contestants' aspirations and desire to look and feel more youthful. So the young–old image is in many ways the ideal body for the forum participants.

In the following example, an online forum participant brings to light how the programme depicts ordinary programme participants as victims of their class and social environments as well as their ageing bodies. The viewer states that *10 Years Younger in 10 Days* involves:

> A bunch of superficial so called fashion experts from the inner city poking fun at not so well kept people from the bush. I just imagine them sitting in some trendy cafe in Sydney's Paddington with a new couple to work on – 'Errrrr your not from around here are you darlings?' I wonder if they have bitch sessions about the people they work on. 'Errrrr his teeth are so revulting!' or 'Get me out of here I will not be seen on television with such a repulsive person' (Westender, 2009).

It is well documented that reality television is equated with universalising middle-class values, behaviour and taste (Kendall cited in Gray, 2008, p. 159; Ringrose & Walkerdine, 2008; Wood & Skeggs, 2008). Working-class lives on television are often depicted as devoid of middle-class values and progressive approaches to lifestyle. Helen Wood and Bev Skeggs (p. 187) explain that 'modes of everyday life are often turned into spectacles of shame', they note how the British *10 Years Younger* presents smoking, sun worshipping and poor diet as reckless and reprehensible. Whereas the focus of the British version may have been directly on class differences, the Australian version is somewhat camouflaged – it focuses on lifestyle, work and family roles, which nevertheless add up to class distinctions.

Confronting Ageing with 10 Years Younger in 10 Days?

Some online viewers query the accuracy of the public's assessments of programme contestants' ages and, by doing so, reveal how the public gaze essentializes age. One online viewer exclaims, '58, seriously?! Have they seen people in their 50s?? It was so contrived' (inhershoes, 2009). However, this viewer's comment implies that a person's age can be determined visually. This view is emulated by many other forum participants. Other online viewers were also critical of the age estimates made by members of the public in the show – their criticisms suggest that signs of ageing are cultural, and that collectively, we ought to be wary about how signs are decoded.

Furthermore, oldness is signified in *10 Years Younger in 10 Days* through obvious physical markers such as contestants' clothing, body weight, skin texture, hair colour and volume. Primarily, the show assumes that 'looking bad' is equated with being old and, as a consequence, looking old is undesirable (Coupland, 2009). On television programmes such as this the young–old is endorsed as the norm. The desire to look younger than one's chronological years is presented as a universal aspiration, fulfilling such an aspiration justifies significant financial outlay to purchase plastic surgery and beauty products (Coupland, 2009; Ringrose & Walkerdine, 2008). One online viewer ruefully comments on the programme's assumptions:

> I must admit the show is something different – it's not often you see real everyday people being served the cold hard facts that they are OLD and UGLY on national television – every single aspect of their bodies pointed out and criticised. Then, in good humour, surgery is suggested to 'return them to their youth', albeit a plastic looking one in the absence of nature (gooseball, 2009).

As contestants' older bodies look more youthful they are imprisoned in two ways. It appears that the first prison for most of the contestants is the emotional and psychological one, where they are imprisoned through their own self-beliefs and their desire to look more youthful. Once contestants take on board the styling, grooming and cosmetic surgery, their prison takes the form of obsessing about their looks and subjecting themselves to the surveillance of the grooming and personal training experts, and people in the public realm. Thus persevering to try and attain the ideal young–old body requires psychological as well as physical energy and the ability to pay for surgery, products and clothing.

However, at the time of the show's release in 2009, some audience members refuted the universal assumption that ageing is undesirable, and not all audience members identified with the programme's assumptions about ageing. For instance, Wendy Harmer, writing for *The Age*, describes *10 Years Younger in 10 Days* as '*Backyard Blitz* for humans'. She observes that, like fairy tales, makeover shows 'infantilise us and keep us from the deeper psychological challenges of confronting ageing' (2009). Marieke Hardy in *The Age* notes *10 Years Younger in 10 Days'* failure to engage with the diversity of ageing when she proclaims, 'I don't want to chase the elusive dream of youth and the superficial idea that to be beautiful one must resemble Gwyneth Paltrow' (2009). Whereas Hardy claims to have been aged by watching 'something as poisonous as *10 Years Younger in 10 Days*', Harmer reflects on the desire to eradicate '10 good years of child-rearing and honest work' from contestants' faces and on television's ability to make this desire seem 'heart-warming'. Both reviewers centre on the way the television programme frames ageing as something to be disparaged.

Sonia Kruger, frames the programme's angle about ageing in her quips, such as 'So much work, so little time' (Episode 1) and rhetorical questions such as 'It seems the older we get, the faster we age and there's not much we can do about it, or is there?' (Episode 5). Online participants saw Kruger and some of the stylists' comments as 'mean', 'rude', 'irritating', 'fake', 'patronizing' and 'inappropriate' (fashion.forward26, 2009; MagickalGoddess, 2009; Maria-TheGourmetChallenge, 2009; ~nareen~, 2009; roe, 2009; unquisite, 2009). Others commented 'What a horrible and mean-spirited show. I certainly won't watch it again' (Shiny, 2009). The attitudes of the stylists and experts towards the makeover contestants were also seen as patronizing. Online participant Meg_Bellamy comments:

> And that disgusting hairdresser – 'there's no such thing as natural beauty'. PLEASE. Way to make people feel even more ugly and like they need to BUY more products. Not watching again! (2009).

Other online forum participants also expressed empathy as well as sympathy for some contestants who were belittled by Kruger and/or members of the style team.

The Use of Cosmetic Surgery

Extreme Makeover, *Nip/Tuck*, *The Swan*, *I Want a Famous Face*, *10 Years Younger* and *Brand New You* are television shows that involve makeover transformations – each programme includes cosmetic surgery in its suite of makeovers. Moreover, programmes like *Extreme Makeover* promote invasive cosmetic surgery. According to Featherstone (2010, p. 203), *Extreme Makeover* is the first reality television programme to feature glamour transformations of ordinary people using cosmetic surgery, and present this surgery as accessible to the average person (also see Franco, 2008). The programme chooses people to be given a Hollywood style makeover, which involves invasive plastic surgery, laser eye surgery, cosmetic dentistry, hairstyling, makeup artistry and fitness. Featherstone (2010) notes that the American Society for Aesthetic Plastic Surgery estimates there has been a 44 per cent increase in the total number of cosmetic procedures since *Extreme Makeover* began in 2002.

10 Years Younger in 10 Days, albeit to a much lesser extent, also features cosmetic surgery as a viable procedure. However, the treatments are often limited to eye lifts, face lifts, Botox and fillers. Some of the online participants on *Vogue's* discussion forum draw attention to the use of such procedures on the show. They compare the show to invasive surgical makeover shows such as *The Swan* and *Extreme Makeover* and generally express disappointment about the inclusion of cosmetic options. Especially disappointing to online viewers is that surgery is given equal weight to other, less invasive and potentially more valuable, strategies and techniques, such as diet, health, grooming, fashion, lifestyle, and wellbeing. In these comments, online viewers explicitly reject the programme's use of cosmetic procedures to reinvent the ageing body:

> The thing I hate about all these type of shows is they just make everyone look the same. Everyone gets the same shape eyes, the big lips, the plump cheeks and obvious chin … I hate how they take away the lines on everyone's faces. We are meant to have lines! I hate it. I like everyone looking different and unique – it's so much more interesting to look at! (karol, 2009).

> Disappointing .. thought it was going to about teaching ppl how to better care for themselves, fashion/health and lifestyle tips not this is how you fork out $$ to get some surgeon to make you look younger. Poor form Chan 7 (MissFlick, 2009).

> Didn't like the comment this week of 'we are going to make you look beautiful'. Completely different attitude to that of Trinny & Sussanah or Carson where it is more about embracing and learning to love the body you are in. I find those shows far more inspirational (lozz, 2009).

The comments above endorse the idea that ageing and how one looks is an individual process and should not be standardized or given over to a commercial nondescript style. For one online participant, 'They turned two normal people into hollywood plastics with cheesy grins. So fake' (nescafed, 2009).

From the *Vogue* online audience's point of view, the show would be more appealing if it focused on showing people what looks good on them at any age:

> ETA my observation is always that nice teeth and a good haircut and some decent clothes make a massive difference to people's appearance. They don't even need all that surgery, usually (karol, 2009).

> Exactly. Just a haircut would have cut ten years off the guy. Probably won't watch this again (jeschique, 2009).

> I didn't realise this was about cosmetic surgery either. Kinda disappointing, I thought it would be about health, clothes, grooming etc. (missmelba, 2009).

> Same, i thought it was going to be 'Queer Eye For The Straight Guy' meets 'What Not To Wear' with a bit of 'You Are What You Eat' and just a touch of Oprah's remembering your spirit!!! (pink lipgloss, 2009).

> I love these types of shows but this fell short. Trinny & Susannah Undress is a million times better. No plastic surgery, a lot better wardrobe choices and they actually deal with the emotional issues behind the couple's problems, instead of just focusing on superficial aspects. It is really good. I thought they looked good at the end but a little try-hard … the hat was too much, and I did not think her outfit was very classy. I liked her hair but I think that it was obvious that his was dyed. I think the show is tacky (fashionista_89, 2009).

While online viewers generally do not agree with the idea of surgically removing physical signs of ageing, they do express a yearning to manage the ageing body. The young–old image lies beneath many comments made by online viewers. On the *Vogue* forum, criticisms of cosmetic procedures suggest this online community support the idea of growing old in conjunction with the physical changes of the ageing body, yet, at the same time, they agree that individuals ought to use techniques – apart from cosmetic surgery – to avoid looking physically old. Thus, online audiences indicate that television has a role to play in assisting viewers to style themselves as they grow older – for this reason, they want to see programmes give advice about grooming, clothing and wellbeing, whatever the age. Online participants highlight here a particularly important disabling social attitude – namely that individuals can maintain the young–old look if they fully participate in a consumer culture.

The Final Unveil: Positive Ageing and the Young–Old

In the closing segment when the participants reveal their new look, the programme prioritizes the physical outward show of youthfulness. For instance, Julie, one participant in the programme, comments:

> Looking young is fantastic, but to feel younger is just as important. We hope we can both do this because we want to start our lives again. We'll get back to what we were hopefully when we were twenty. [Julie looks at her reflection in the mirror and smooths the skin on her neck.] Bit of a blast from the past, but that's what it will be like. I hope he takes one look at me and just loves it (Episode 8).

Here Julie alludes to how the makeover goes some way to mending the fractured self through restoring the body so it looks more youthful. For the presenter, the contestants' routines and family bonds have created an old body – inside of which there is an authentic, youthful self longing to be revived. In short, it suggests that there is an inner being wrestling with the ageing body.

However, while this trope epitomizes the possibility of contestants reclaiming their youthful selves, the programme risks encasing the ageing body in surface images (Gailey, 2007). Contestants are under pressure from the presenter and experts in *10 Years Younger in 10 Days* to achieve personal goals consistent with their own authentic self, yet, contestants are made-over from the experts' standpoint. The programme's focus on the inner authentic self trapped in the ageing bodies is used to justify the use of cosmetic procedures to change the outer older body to look closer in age to the internal self. As Heyes explains, the use of cosmetic procedures in the context of makeover programmes 'is less about becoming *beautiful*', it is 'more about becoming *oneself*', which means contestants developing the capabilities and aptitudes that were beyond them in the past (2007, p. 96).

Conclusion

Television media attempts to essentialize and quantify old age, even though old age cannot be defined just by physical appearance or chronology. Old age is a cultural construct, and the context of ageing should be considered rather than old age as a discrete category (Degnen, 2007; Vesperi, 1985). We have argued that television programmes that try to quantify old age disregard the context in which characters or participants are ageing, and we have provided samples of online audiences referring to this problem in their discussion of *10 Years Younger in 10 Days*.

Ultimately television persists in shoring up essentialized notions of what it means to be old. In addition, depictions of ageing on television continue to be informed by dominant discourses such as that old age is a state of decline and that positive ageing means successfully overcoming the impediments of old age. Yet televisual depictions of ageing have recently begun to change with older people being represented as more active, as socially engaged, as mentally astute, as physically healthy, and as pursuing meaningful work. On today's television, active and youthful older people or characters are being touted as the standard to reach. Our discussion of *Hot in Cleveland* as well as *10 Years Younger in 10 Days* reveals the elements that support the new norm – the rise of a consumer culture, current research and biomedical advances (Bradley & Longino, 2001, p. 18; see Featherstone & Wernick, 1995).

As can be seen from the discussion above, online viewers and participants tended to disidentify with most of the *10 Years Younger in 10 Days* participants. From our viewpoint, a major reason this occurred is because the programme's techniques encourage audience disidentification with the ageing body. One way this disidentification occurs is through the producer's perpetuation of familiar binaries such as young/old, city/country, groomed/ungroomed and fashionable/unfashionable. However, programme makers, participants and online viewers identify with the need to manage the visible ageing body because looking physically old is deemed undesirable.

Chapter 8
Conclusion: Beyond the Water-Cooler – Reinforcing and Contesting the Symbolic Annihilation of Disability, Obesity and Ageing

> Now there is no question they are aware and that they are aware of our engagement with the show and support of the lack of weight loss focus. When the creators, producers, writers, actors, and anyone else receives pressure to promote weight loss or play to the weight loss crowd, we might give them extra reason to resist. Given that they seem to have a bit of a predisposition to resist, we might have a goddamned chance here. Now, weight loss companies are powerful, but we are powerful too (withoutscene, 2010).

The television shows discussed throughout this book have had an unquestionable influence on the representation of disability, obesity and ageing on popular television today. They also draw on a long history of the cultural negation of these groups. Each programme selected for analysis in this book, whether *The Biggest Loser*, *Grumpy Old Men* or even the lesser known, *Packed to the Rafters*, has also elicited an energetic online discussion (or tele-participation) from both ordinary viewers and social activists.

These discussions constitute a culturally significant, ongoing and open-ended body of work for both media researchers and television audiences. Both the social activist movements and the online viewers' discussions are a principal resource in this book for gauging the reception of televisual portrayals of disability, obesity and ageing. In addition, these discussions offer insights beyond a reflection of public attitudes because they constitute a text themselves that can be read in concert with the televisual representation. Unlike water-cooler conversations, insights posted online become texts that can be referred back to by people engaging with a process of meaning making. These discussions do more than operate in parallel to televisual depictions – they become part of the media world of meaning making. As we have argued throughout this book, the television media world now extends beyond programme makers and the networks to include online audiences.

In this concluding chapter we draw together the issues and arguments that percolate throughout this book. These arguments are pivotal to our doing a cross-genre analysis of disability, obesity and ageing portrayals in televisual media.

Television Entertainment: Framing Marginalization

Throughout this book we have followed the work of Jonathan Gray. Gray (2008) explores the impacts of television entertainment – including the broadcast text and the overflow onto online platforms – on our daily lives and the ways we think about marginalized groups. As we discussed in Chapters 2 and 3, online audiences often examine televisual representations of disability, obesity and ageing in the context of reality. Although we recognize that realism is itself a construction on television, television does indeed frame reality as Gray suggests by influencing the ways we think about certain groups, such as the disabled, old and obese. This reality can also be contaminated by repetitive televisual representation (p. 121). According to Couldry's (2002) theory of symbolic power, if a particular image of disability, obesity and ageing is constantly repeated on television then this image becomes the public's perception of this group. Throughout this book we have argued the question of whether programmes encourage audiences to seek out reality or to replace it with fiction or untruths is particularly important to ask when analysing the televisual construction of marginalized groups such as people who are disabled, older or obese. As such we have analysed the ways online audiences respond to the fictions and untruths presented in television texts. Although television offers exposure to people that may exist outside our immediate frame of reference, it can also adopt a normative formula to marginalize them further.

Online audiences engage with this process of analysis by thinking about representations and responding to them, especially in terms of marginalization. Online audiences comment on or criticize the way programme makers marginalize particular characters or contestants because of their body size, disability or age. From this perspective, the online conversations we include are not just negotiations, but negotiations around specific realities based on identifications and disidentifications with disability, obesity and ageing. The responses are nuanced and varied, because sometimes they are negotiations, but at other times they focus on what audiences like or find disgusting etc. By contesting what is on television, online audiences point to the representational limits of media depictions, and, at the same time, they draw attention to the potential for their revision.

This so-called tele-participation allows audiences to move from a generalized experience of television that broadcasts to a universal audience to the formation of communities of interest with other online audiences and social movement activists. One of our concerns in this book has been the ways television reception is being changed and shaped by what Williams (2009, p. 43) calls 'collective intelligence'. In Chapters 4 and 5 we gave samples of how topics about disabilities and bullying are being discussed on official and unofficial forums, social movement sites, talkback radio, and blogger sites. These online communities, bounded by common interests, enable viewers to discuss, contest and challenge their and others' televisual experiences.

Whereas television is saturated with images of acceptable bodies that ascribe to culturally sanctioned notions of normality, often our own bodies do not measure up to these representations. Fat and disabled bodies take on a particular significance in this obsession because cultural prejudice has long dictated that disabled bodies must be cured. This imperative, to intervene and cure, is now being applied to obese bodies. Old age is similarly seen in the popular zeitgeist as a condition best avoided or at a minimum addressed with specialized intervention. Yet social context decides what is considered old, fat or disabled, with nuanced definitions needed in different cultural contexts.

Contesting Media Discourses

Throughout this book we argued that contesting media discourses about disability, obesity and ageing in public forums is a significant activity for audiences and viewers. When we first began researching this book, we thought that attitudes towards and depictions of disability, obesity and ageing on television would be similar. We considered these groups to be amongst the most loathed and feared identifications in society. We hypothesized that the portrayals would include the usual narrow repertoires such as excessive or grotesque bodies, characters in minor roles and unrepresentable bodies no-one wants to see on television. We thought that online audiences would respond to depictions of disability, obesity and old age in similar, if not identical, ways.

Although we noticed similarities in the televisual portrayals of disability, obesity and ageing such as characters in each of the categories being mostly in minor roles, often subjected to disabling attitudes, and depicted as bodies out of control, we discovered that online audiences have responded to the images in diverse ways. For instance, with the exception of activists, we found online audiences rarely identify as disabled or old; however, several identified as obese. Similarly, ageing activists do not exist in significant numbers, with ageing audiences largely coming online to discuss favourite characters and storylines. Whereas online viewers' responses to portrayals of disability, obesity and ageing have been varied, both the disability and fat acceptance movements constantly find fault with nearly all the televisual representations. Public discussion on all the forums cited in this book offer a *window* into cultural conceptions of visual images about the normative and non-normative body.

We have drawn on the social model of disability throughout this book to connect televisual representations of disability, obesity and ageing. People who are disabled, obese and old, along with experiencing possible bodily limitations are disempowered by inflexible social practices, and prejudicial attitudes, images and narratives that see these bodies as inferior. Thus, we used the term disabling social attitudes to group these identifications together as similarly subjugated identities. While approaching the generally subjugated position of each identification, individual chapters of this book reveal a different focus – disability is explored in terms of normality, with analysis of ageing revealing problematic gender representations, while obesity draws on the health costs to the nation. Although online audiences may medicalize all three, disability bloggers proceed from a social model to highlight social disablement and seniors writers tend to operate within the paradigm of an affirmation model to celebrate perceived positive representations. Fat acceptance writers by comparison move between the social and affirmation models.

Yet particular understandings about disability, obesity and ageing are validated on television and made to appear *normal*, whereas others are constructed as marginal and/or aberrant. For example, social movement responses to institutional discourse (whether medical or media) are often judged as spurious and lacking credibility. One example of a marginalized perspective is the fat acceptance movement's idea of 'health at every size' (O'Hara, 2008). On ABC (Australia), *The Drum Opinion* online forum, Lily O'Hara representing the movement elaborates:

> In recent years, a new idea about weight has emerged. It is called the Health at Every Size (HAES) paradigm and it moves the focus away from the weight loss-to-be-healthy model. Developed in the United States and increasingly embraced by the fat acceptance movement, HAES argues that a person's ideal weight cannot be measured by the scales or mathematical equations such as body mass index. It teaches that we should respect and appreciate the rich diversities of body shapes and sizes.

However, other online audiences writing in response, on *The Drum Opinion* deemed the fat acceptance view aberrant, and few endorsed O'Hara's perspective, except for Catherine (2009) who comments:

> Well having read all 334 comments I still haven't found fault with Lily's article. Interestingly only a few of you have picked up on what Lily is actually saying in

> her article and what the HAES philosophy actually is. We are so programmed now to react to fat with horror and disgust that the mere mention of the word brings on incredibly strong opinions as is clearly demonstrated here. God help someone who challenges the traditional weight focused health paradigm and who dares to suggest that perhaps we should shift the focus to wellbeing instead of weight? For all who may bother to read this far, the message from Lily is very clear and intelligent. There are countless studies to show that diets do not work.

Throughout the book we have given examples of stereotypes that the televisual media circulate. Many of these stereotypes, through over-use by television writers, become 'regressive depictions' in the form of 'archetypes' (Gray, 2008, p. 106). They are loaded with meaning and offer clear semiotic and narrative shortcuts. For instance, the character with a disability is represented as either inspirational or tragic (for example participants with disabilities on reality television); the person who is fat is shown overeating (for example, participants in *The Biggest Loser*, 2012) to validate why they are lonely and loveless; the character who is old is shown in a nursing home or hospital (for example in *Getting On*) which becomes shorthand for a declining body close to death. These stereotypes become integrated into the tacit knowledge that viewers draw on regarding these groups. In many cases, viewers are unaware that such depictions are stereotypes even when naming people they know who do not fit the stereotype (Philo et al., 1994).

Structures of Power

Throughout the book we have called attention to the structures of power that shape television representation – in particular, the power of television networks to frame, shape and store the images they circulate. Television institutions compete with each other to increase ratings and to sell programmes – these competing interests shore up televisual power. Often television networks exercise control over writers and creators of programmes (see the documentary *America in Primetime*, 2011; Gillan, 2011) in their endeavour to woo advertisers. Even though contesting discourses do emerge on television, researchers and viewers need to be mindful of who claims authority to speak.

Television production techniques tend to amplify and legitimate particular voices – alternative voices that contest the media discourse become 'invisible' (Tang & Yang, 2011, p. 677). What is in the media limelight gains attention, what is not is symbolically annihilated and/or treated as insignificant (cf. Tuchman, 1978). For instance, in the case of obesity, certain ways of speaking about obese people, such as the type of food and the quantity they eat, are made audible and visible. Whereas, the medical conditions and genetics that increase weight are frequently concealed or ignored on television.

In an increasingly media-saturated society, people are both more subject to 'ideal' images about the body and more aware of how unnatural and unfair these are (Wolf, 2002, pp. 3–7). For instance, in Chapter 7 online audiences discussing *10 Years Younger in 10 Days* point to how the programme presenters and experts pressure contestants to reach an ideal body image that was contrary to their rural lifestyles. Other online audiences highlight how presenters and experts persuade contestants on makeover programmes, such as *The Swan* and *Extreme Makeover: Weight Loss Edition*, to have cosmetic surgery in order to attain a body ideal that is beyond most people's body makeup and financial resources.

Cultural Ideals

Indeed many online audiences cling to the value that characters or participants can and should control their body and work towards meeting the 'ideal' standard (Wendell, 1996, p. 89). Thus, televisual media offers audiences a 'cultural ideal' that constantly raises the 'standard of normality' (Snyder & Mitchell, 2010; Wendell, 1996, p. 89). Yet this is a standard that is very difficult if not impossible to meet for most viewers. To be seen in control of one's body requires contestants, participants and audiences to engage in *masquerades* of normality.

However, for many people just 'falling within the "normal" range is not enough', often they are persuaded and 'pressured' to 'try to meet the ideal' (Wendell, 1996, p. 89). This ideal standard, as Snyder and Mitchell (2010, p. 187) identify, becomes the 'target' of genres that focus on bodies – these programmes reinforce the 'fantasy of bodily control' among audience and viewers. Those who are unable to control their disability, weight or frailty are rejected on television – their bodies fall well short of the normal standard.

We have suggested throughout this book that televisual depictions of characters and participants who are disabled, old and obese pose a threat to the audiences regarding their tenuous control over their own bodies. That said, these representations may also be used to make audiences *feel better* about themselves. For instance, in Chapter 4 we discussed how Susan Boyle in the audition of *Britain's Got Talent* was constructed as an unattractive, slightly overweight and frumpy contestant – someone who most viewers did not want to identify with. Yet she seemed to make people feel better about their own self-perceived inadequate bodies, lives and careers. In Gray's words, (2008, p. 121) television can make us 'feel better about ourselves', by providing depictions of others who fall below the minimum standards of normality – that is, those whose behaviour is considered abnormal, those who have physical weaknesses, and those whose body size is deemed large. Of course all of us, including those who fall short of meeting the minimum standard, are subject to 'disciplinary practices of physical normality' (Wendell, 1996, p. 88); these practices create a standard of normality against which ordinary people measure themselves. Online audiences can now participate in discussions about these standards, which does not mean the standard of measurement disappears or no longer exists. However, through discussants' identifications and disidentifications the norm can be questioned, challenged and negotiated.

The focus in this book has been on online audience activity, that is, how audiences *use* official-generated and unofficial-generated television websites which discuss disability, obesity and ageing. In our case studies in Chapters 5, 6 and 7, we found that identification, disidentification and negotiation inform online viewers' use of various modes of expression to perform their identities within the online forum setting. Through the act of identifying or disidentifying with characters and participants on television, online audiences regularly negotiate and avert what could be described as disabling televisual imagery in the context of representations of disability, obesity and ageing.

Dis/Identification

Identification is a key feature of our analysis. Often online audiences reveal emotional and fleeting identification with characters and participants as ordinary people participating in the media world. However, as revealed in the online viewers' comments in each of the chapters, these processes of identifying and disidentifying are not opposites, 'rather they occupy two sides of an emotional triangle' (de Swaan, 1997, p. 106; Medina, 2003, p. 659). Indeed, people must first identify in order to disidentify. Yet online audiences are repeatedly oblivious to this 'cognitive distancing' (Elsbach & Battacharya, 2001, p. 399). Many online viewers perceive that the identity of a disabled, fat or old character is too distant from themselves. Thus, viewers may or may not reject identities that resemble themselves, choosing to evaluate contestants and characters against the standard body type by which all individuals are measured – that is, the norm which as we have discussed is morphing with the ideal. So, some online discussions actually intensify the affect of disabling imagery, and, as a consequence, perpetuate television's symbolic power and the symbolic annihilation of disability, obesity and ageing.

Much of the discursive and audience research in media and cultural studies has focused on examining and articulating how the media depict gender, sexuality, race and class. Therefore, disability, obesity and ageing are relatively new concerns. We have investigated these identity categories in concert as rejected bodies because each is culturally moulded and subjected to disabling social attitudes. Too often, the depiction of disabled, obese and old age identities on television are essentialized. What's more, discussants in the official-generated and viewer-generated sites frequently perpetuate the social attitude that being disabled, obese or old is abnormal. Thus, discussants' views deepen the stigma attached to these identities. Equally however, these online spaces provide the opportunity to contest television's symbolic power.

By alerting other viewers to framing and editing techniques programme makers use, it is clear that online audience members often doubt and question claims made on television. From that perspective, viewers were often self-reflexive about their own participation and use of programmes. Yet, even when online audiences were aware of the way television shapes particular portrayals of disability, obesity and ageing, they may be oblivious to certain disabling attitudes.

The focus of our book has been on whether audiences *identify* with the characters, situations and storylines about disability, obesity and old age offered on television. Although online discussions do veer towards describing some representations as positive and others negative, some as realistic, others as unrealistic, our analysis reveals that online audiences' responses do not fall neatly into any of these two camps. We conclude that online discourse is an important site of cultural mediation. Our efforts to analyse the three case studies have brought us to the realization that we, and other researchers, need to deepen our examination of diversity in televisual media, and our consideration of what this might mean for how non-normative groups are represented.

Throughout this book we have critiqued representations that symbolically annihilate disability, obesity and ageing on television. However, we are hopeful also and have indeed alluded to representations and discussions that recognize and celebrate the increasingly diverse ways these groups are being shown on television and online media. Thus we look to the future with optimism. There is enormous potential for the online environment to contribute to discourses of disability, obesity and ageing by providing a greater diversity through the mobilization of social justice movements around these identities.

It has been beyond the scope of this book to question what actual impact online forums have on television production and media representations. Whereas withoutscene (2010) cited at the head of the chapter believes online discussion offers a feedback loop to television producers who are listening, we are not as certain. We do, however, hope that these online conversations develop a threshold of consciousness of the social disablement of disability, obesity and ageing. This is a vital area of future research.

References

20Valvetop. (2012, May 14). Re: The Voice Australia: Darren v Brett [Online forum comment]. Retrieved from http://www.youtube.com/all_comments?threaded=1&v=E0PZuDbLY6U

73yearsyoung. (2005, May 5). Re: Television [Online forum comment]. Retrieved from http://www.seniors.gov.au/internet/seniors/meetingplace/main.nsf/topiccontributions?Open&ID=E5A061C81A0BCC76CA256FC7007B1B30&Start=21&

Abbyjean. (2009, December 16). Transcontinental Disability Choir: 9021-Oh No! [Online review]. Retrieved from http://bitchmagazine.org/post/transcontinental-disability-choir-9021-oh-no

ABC message board. (n.d.). Retrieved from http://www2b.abc.net.au/tmb/Client/MessageBoardList.aspx?g=44

About. (n.d.). FWD (Feminists with Disability) for a way forward [Online forum]. Retrieved from http://disabledfeminists.com/about/

About us. (n.d.). AARP, who we are, what we do, what guides us. Retrieved from http://www.aarp.org/about-aarp/

Actionmage. (2011, May 4). Re: Television without pity: Mike & Molly [Online forum comment]. Retrieved from http://forums.televisionwithoutpity.com/index.php?showtopic=3198677&st=330

Adele04. (2009, April 22). Re: Ch 7's '10 Years Younger in 10 Days' [Online forum comment]. Retrieved from http://forums.vogue.com.au/showthread.php?t=329712&page=3

Alison. (2009, September 4). I have another confession … [Web log post]. Retrieved from http://thinkingofstartingablog.blogspot.com.au/2009_09_01_archive.html

almitywife. (2009, January 22). Re: Are we all sadistic sickos? [Online forum comment]. Retrieved from http://community.ten.com.au/community/the_biggest_loser

Andrejevic, M. (2004). *Reality TV: The work of being watched.* Lanham, MA: Rowman & Littlefield Publishers.

Andrejevic, M. (2008). Watching Television Without Pity: The productivity of online fans. *Television & New Media, 9*(1), 24-46.

Anonymous. (2009, October 2). Re: I have another confession [Web log comment]. Retrieved from http://thinkingofstartingablog.blogspot.com.au/2009/09/i-have-another-confession.html

Arboleda, S. (2010, July 2). 'Huge' offers a realistic portrayal of overweight teens [Web log post]. Retrieved from http://zeldalily.com/index.php/2010/07/huge-offers-a-realistic-portrayal-of-overweight-teens/

Arnold Ward. (2010, October 28). Re: Internet outrage over 'bigoted' *Marie Claire* blog (posted by former anorexic) that criticises 'fat people making out on TV' [Online forum comment]. Retrieved from http://www.dailymail.co.uk/news/article-1324373/Are-cool-fat-people-making-TV-Marie-Claire-blog-post-anorexic-causes-internet-uproar.html#ixzz2EFopoL6Q

ASPEN. (2010, February 4). Re: New reality show: I'm Hotter Than My Daughter on Sodahead [Online forum comment]. Retrieved from http://www.sodahead.com/entertainment/new-reality-show-im-hotter-than-my-daughter/blog-253001/?q=Hotter%20than%20my%20Daughter%20on%20Sodahead&page=2#comments

Austral ®. (2010, August 3). Re: Grumpy Old Women Friday evenings late [Online forum comment]. Retrieved from http://www2b.abc.net.au/tmb/Client/PrintFriendlyMessage.aspx?b=81&m=90896

autostradas. (2011, May 2). Re: TV review: Vera and Exile [Online forum comment]. Retrieved from http://www.guardian.co.uk/tv-and-radio/2011/may/01/tv-review-vera-exile#comment-10573237

Banting, W. (1863). Letter of corpulence. Retrieved from http://www.thefitblog.net/ebooks/LetterOnCorpulence/LetteronCorpulence.pdf

Barnes, C. (1992). *Disabling imagery and the media: An exploration of the principles for media representations of disabled people.* Report for the British Council of Organisations of Disabled People. Retrieved from http://www.leeds.ac.uk/disability-studies/archiveuk/Barnes/disabling%20imagery.pdf

Barnes, C. (1997). A legacy of oppression: A history of disability in Western culture. In L. Barton & M. Oliver (Eds.), *Disability studies: Past present and future* (pp. 3-24). Leeds: The Disability Press.

Barnes, C. (2004). Disability, disability studies and the humanities. In J. Swain, S. French, C. Barnes & C. Thomas (Eds.), *Disabling barriers – enabling environments* (pp. 28-33). Los Angeles: SAGE.

bartybates. (2009, May 4). Re: 10 Years Younger in 10 Days [Online forum comment]. Retrieved from http://forums.whirlpool.net.au/archive/1195197

Basting, A. D. (1998). *The stages of age: Performing age in contemporary American culture.* Ann Arbor, MI: University of Michigan Press.

Bastow, C. (2009, September 24). Australian television's disability tension [Web log post]. Retrieved from http://www.thevine.com.au/entertainment/blogs/australian-televisions-disability-tension/

Bastow, C. (2011, September 2). Disability on the small screen: What's wrong with this picture? [Web log post]. Retrieved from http://www.abc.net.au/rampup/articles/2011/09/02/3308488.htm

beetle. (2005, July 15). Re: Television. Meeting place: Television [Online forum comment]. Retrieved from http://www.seniors.gov.au/internet/seniors/meetingplace/main.nsf/topiccontributions?Open&ID=E5A061C81A0BCC76CA256FC7007B1B30&Start=11&

Bell, J. (1992). In search of a discourse on aging: The elderly on television. *The Gerontologist, 32*(3), 305-311.

Big Brother Little Sister. (2009, September 4). Re: I have another confession … [Web log comment]. Retrieved from http://thinkingofstartingablog.blogspot.com.au/2009/09/i-have-another-confession.html

Big Fat Blog. (n.d.). Retrieved from http://www.bigfatblog.com/

Big Fat Blog. (2010, November 3). BFB's virtual kiss-in!!! [Web log post]. Retrieved from http://www.bigfatblog.com/bfbs-virtual-kiss

Bilt4Cmfrt. (2010, June 29). Re: HUGE mistake [Web log comment]. Retrieved from http://www.bigfatblog.com/huge-mistake

Bogdan, R. (1990). *Freak show: Presenting human oddities for amusement and profit.* Chicago: University of Chicago Press.

bonnie. (2005, May 15). Re: Television [Online forum comment]. Retrieved from http://www.seniors.gov.au/internet/seniors/meetingplace/main.nsf/topiccontributions?Open&ID=E5A061C81A0BCC76CA256FC7007B1B30&Start=21&

Bourdieu, P. (1991). *Language and symbolic power* (G. Raymond & M. Adamson, Trans.). Oxford: Polity Press.

Bradley, D. E., & Longino, C. F. (2001). How older people think about images of aging in advertising and the media. *Generations, 25*(3), 17-21.

Brandon, T., & Pritchard, G. (2011). 'Being fat': A conceptual analysis using three models of disability. *Disability & Society, 26*(1), 79-92.

Bratich, J. Z. (2007). Programming reality: Control societies, new subjects and the powers of transformation. In D. A. Heller (Ed.), *Makeover television: Realities remodelled* (pp. 6-22). London: I.B. Tauris.

brideofhorror. (2009, February 24). Re: tbl and eating is it just me? [Online forum comment]. Retrieved from http://community.ten.com.au/community/the_biggest_loser

Britain's Missing Top Model (n.d.). Retrieved from http://www.bbc.co.uk/programmes/b00cfhhb

Brooker, W. (2004). Living on *Dawson's Creek*: Teen viewers, cultural convergence, and television overflow. In R. C. Allen & A. Hill (Eds.), *The television studies reader* (pp. 569-580). London: Routledge.

Brown, J. (2011). Britain's missing top model; a feminist perspective [Web log post]. Retrieved from http://www.abc.net.au/rampup/articles/2011/03/09/3159387.htm

Bryant, L., & Pini, B. (2009). Gender, class and rurality: Australian case studies. *Journal of Rural Studies, 25*(1), 48-57.

Butler, J. (1993). *Bodies that matter: On the discursive limits of 'sex'.* New York: Routledge.
Butler, J. (2004). *Precarious life: The powers of mourning and violence.* London: Verso.
Cactusfreek. (2009, February 3). Re: Concerned [Online forum comment]. Retrieved from http://community.ten.com.au/community/the_biggest_loser
CarrieP. (2010, April 30). Living while fat [Web log post]. Retrieved from http://www.bigfatblog.com/living-while-fat
Catherine. (2009, February 18). Re: Fat Acceptance. *The Drum Opinion* [Web log comment]. http://www.abc.net.au/unleashed/32464.html
cathur. (2009, February 23). Re: tbl and eating is it just me? [Online forum comment]. Retrieved from http://community.ten.com.au/community/the_biggest_loser
chipolata. (2010, October 31). Re: The British Comedy Guide [Online forum comment]. Retrieved from http://www.comedy.co.uk/forums
Chivers, S. (2011). *The silvering screen: Old age and disability in cinema.* Toronto: University of Toronto Press.
Chivers, S., & Markotić, N. (Eds.). (2010). *The problem body: Projecting disability on film.* Columbus, OH: Ohio State University Press.
chocifan. (2012, April 3). Re: Selena's bombshell [Online forum comment]. Retrieved from http://www.community.ten.com.au/community/the_biggest_loser
Chory-Assad, R. M., & Yanen, A. (2005). Hopelessness and loneliness as predictors of older adults' involvement with favorite television performers. *Journal of Broadcasting & Electronic Media, 49*(2), 182-201.
Claire. (2009, April 25). Re: Susan Boyle is transforming before our eyes [Web log comment]. Retrieved from http://fresnobeehive.com/archives/2842
Cohen, J. (2001). Defining identification: A theoretical look at the identification of audiences with media characters. *Mass Communication and Society, 4*(3), 246-264.
Cohen, J. (2006). Audience identification with media characters. In J. Bryant & P. Vorderer (Eds.), *Psychology of entertainment* (pp. 183-197). Mahway, NJ: Lawrence Erlbaum.
Comments. (n.d.). Re : Should 'fatties' get a room? (Even on TV?) [Web log comment]. http://www.marieclaire.com/sex-love/dating-blog/overweight-couples-on-television
Contestants. (2012). Selena Brown. Retrieved from http://thebiggestloser.com.au/selena-brown.htm
Costello, V., & Moore, B. (2007). Cultural outlaws: An examination of audience activity and online television fandom. *Television & New Media, 8*(2), 124-143.
Couldry, N. (2000). *The place of media power: Pilgrims and witnesses of the media age.* London: Routledge.

Couldry, N. (2002). Mediation and alternative media, or relocating the centre of media and communication studies. *Media International Australia, Incorporating Culture & Policy, 103*, 24-31.

Coupland, J. (2009). Time, the body and the reversibility of ageing: Commodifying the decade. *Ageing & Society, 29*(6), 953-976.

criketer. (2012, April 3). Re: Selena's bombshell [Online forum comment]. Retrieved from http://www.community.ten.com.au/community/the_biggest_loser

Cristofovici, A. (1999). Touching surfaces: Photography, aging and an aesthetics of change. In K. Woodward (Ed.), *Figuring age: Women, bodies, generations* (pp. 268-293). Bloomington: Indiana University Press.

Cumberbatch, G., & Negrine, R. (1992). *Images of disability on television*. London: Routledge.

Cupcakewa. (2012, March 26). Re: Margie [Online forum comment]. Retrieved from http://community.ten.com.au/community/the_biggest_loser

Darke, P. (1998). Cinematic representations of disability. In T. Shakespeare (Ed.), *The disability reader: Social science perspectives* (pp. 181-200). New York: Continuum.

Darke, P. (2004). The changing face of representations of disability in the media. In J. Swain, S. French, C. Barnes & C. Thomas (Eds.), *Disabling barriers – enabling environments* (pp. 100-105). Los Angeles: SAGE.

David W. (2011, May 21). Re: Vera Review: ITV's drama renaissance continues [Online forum comment]. Retrieved from http://channelhopping.onthebox.com/2011/05/01/vera-review-itvs-drama-renaissance-continues/#comment-83378

DazzleMe. (2012, April 2). Re: Selena's bombshell [Online forum comment]. Retrieved from http://community.ten.com.au/community/the_biggest_loser

DebraSY. (2008, September 23). Toronto Star advice columnist Ellie preaches acceptance [Web log post]. Retrieved from http://www.bigfatblog.com/toronto-star-advice-columnist-ellie-preaches-acceptance

DeeLeigh. (2010, June 29). HUGE Misrepresentation [Web log post]. Retrieved from www.bigfatblog.com/taxonomy/term/19

Deery, J. (2003). TV.com: Participatory viewing on the web. *The Journal of Popular Culture, 37*(2), 161-183.

Degges-White, S., & Myers, J. E. (2006). Women at midlife: An exploration of chronological age, subjective age, wellness, and life satisfaction. *ADULTSPAN, 5*(2), 67-80.

Degnen, C. (2007). Minding the gap: The construction of old age and oldness amongst peers. *Journal of Aging Studies, 21*(1), 69-80.

Deniselle. (2008, March 30). Eating and body image on the Gilmore Girls [Web log post]. Retrieved from http://findingmyvalue.blogspot.com.au/2008/03/eating-and-body-image-on-gilmore-girls.html de Swaan, A. (1997). Widening circles of disidentification: On the psycho- and sociogenesis of the hatred of distant strangers – reflections on Rwanda. *Theory, Culture & Society, 14*(2), 105-122.

Deveny, C. (2009, June 6). You can't gloss over the ugly truth [Online review]. Retrieved from http://www.theage.com.au/articles/2009/06/04/1243708563516.html

DietVader. (2009a, February 19). Re: Degrading and wrong [Online forum comment]. Retrieved from http://community.ten.com.au/community/the_biggest_loser

DietVader. (2009b, February 20). Re: Degrading and wrong [Online forum comment]. Retrieved from http://community.ten.com.au/community/the_biggest_loser

Digital Spy. (n.d.). Retrieved from http://www.digitalspy.com.au/

domesticqueen. (2009, February 23). Re: tbl and eating is it just me? [Online forum comment]. Retrieved from http://community.ten.com.au/community/the_biggest_loser

Donlon, M. M., Ashman, O., & Levy, B. R. (2005). Re-vision of older television characters: A stereotype-awareness intervention. *Journal of Social Issues, 61*(2), 307-319.

dos Santos, K. (2009, November 10). Glee boss gets on board with Puck and Rachel! [Online review]. Retrieved from http://au.eonline.com/news/153052/glee-boss-gets-on-board-with-puck-and-rachel

Dovey, J. (2000). *Freakshow: First person media and factual television.* London: Pluto Press.

Driedger, D. (1989). *The last civil rights movement: Disabled peoples' international.* London: C. Hurst & Co. Publishers.

earle qaeda ®. (2010a, September 18). Re: Australian Programs ABC Message Board – ABC TV Have your say (HYS) [Online forum comment]. Retrieved from http://www2b.abc.net.au/tmb/Client/PrintFriendlyMessage.aspx?b=81&m=95596

earle qaeda ®. (2010b, September 19). Re: Australian Programs ABC Message Board – ABC TV Have your say (HYS) [Online forum comment]. Retrieved from http://www2b.abc.net.au/tmb/Client/PrintFriendlyMessage.aspx?b=81&m=95709

Electrifried. (2009, June 10). Re: 10 Years Younger in 10 Days [Online forum comment]. Retrieved from http://forums.whirlpool.net.au/archive/1195197

Ellis, K. (2008). *Disabling diversity: The social construction of disability in 1990s Australian national cinema.* Saarbrücken, Germany: VDM (Verlag Dr. Müller).

Ellis, K. (2009). A quest through chaos: My narrative of illness and recovery. *Gender Forum: An Internet Journal for Gender Studies, 26*(2). Retrieved from http://www.genderforum.org/issues/literature-and-medicine-ii/a-quest-through-chaos/

Ellis, K., & Goggin, G. (2014). *Disability and the media.* New York: Palgrave Macmillan.

Elsbach, K. D., & Bhattacharya, C. B. (2001). Defining who you are by what you're not: Organizational disidentification and the National Rifle Association. *Organization Science, 12*(4), 393-413.

Elser, D., & Stephenson, A. (2011, February 1). Are we hungry to chew more TV fat? [Online review]. Retrieved from http://www.news.com.au/entertainment/television/are-we-hungry-to-chew-more-tv-fat/story-e6frfmyi-1225998196646

Essential Baby's forums. (2009) Re: Packed to the Rafters [Online forum comments]. Retrieved from http://www.essentialbaby.com.au/forums/lofiversion/index.php/t642685.html

Eyal, K., & Rubin, A. M. (2003). Viewer aggression and homophily, identification, and parasocial relationships with television characters. *Journal of Broadcasting & Electronic Media, 47*(1), 77-98.

Farrell, A. E. (2011). *Fat shame: Stigma and the fat body in American culture.* New York: New York University Press.

fashion.forward26. (2009, April 22). Re: Ch 7's '10 years younger in 10 days' [Online forum comment]. Retrieved from http://forums.vogue.com.au

fashionista_89. (2009, May 6). Re: Ch 7's '10 years younger in 10 days' [Online forum comment]. Retrieved from http://forums.vogue.com.au

Featherstone, M. (2010). Body, image and affect in consumer culture. *Body & Society, 16*(1), 193-221.

Featherstone, M., & Hepworth, M. (1995). Images of positive aging: A case study of *Retirement Choice* magazine. In M. Featherstone & A. Wernick (Eds.), *Images of aging: Cultural representations of later life* (pp. 29-47). London: Routledge.

Featherstone, M., & Wernick, A. (1995). Introduction. In M. Featherstone, & A. Wernick (Eds.), *Images of aging: Cultural representations of later life* (pp. 1-15). London: Routledge.

Finkelstein, R., QC. (2012). *Report of the independent inquiry into the media and media regulation.* Department of Broadband, Communication and the Digital Economy, Australian Government. Retrieved from http://www.archive.dbcde.gov.au/__data/assets/pdf_file/0017/147005/Media-statement-Ray-Finkelstein-QC.pdf

Fishman, T. C. (2010). *Shock of gray: The aging of the world's population and how it pits young against old, child against parent, worker against boss, company against rival, and nation against nation.* New York: Scribner.

Fiske, J., Hodge, B., & Turner, G. (1987). *Myths of Oz: Reading Australian popular culture.* Sydney: Allen & Unwin.

Foucault, M. (1977). *Language, counter-memory, practice: Selected essays and interviews* (S. Simon & D. F. Bouchard, Trans.). Oxford: Blackwell.

Foucault, M. (2005). *The hermeneutics of the subject: Lectures at the Collège de France, 1981–1982* (1st ed.). (G. Burchell, Trans.). New York: Palgrave-Macmillan.

Fouts, G., & Burggraf, K. (2000). Television situation comedies: Female weight, male negative references, and audience reactions. *Sex Roles*, *42*(9/10), 925-932.

Fouts, G., & Vaughan, K. (2002). Television situation comedies: Male weight, negative references, and audience reactions. *Sex Roles*, *46*(11/12), 439-442.

Franco, J. (2008). Extreme Makeover: The politics of gender, class and cultural identity. *Television & New Media*, *9*(6), 471-486.

Fraser, K. (2007). 'Now I am ready to tell how bodies are changed into different bodies … ' Ovid, *The Metamorphoses*. In D. A. Heller (Ed.), *Makeover television: Realities remodelled* (pp. 177-192). London: I.B. Tauris.

Frequently asked questions. (n.d.). The Biggest Loser official forum. Retrieved from http://thebiggestloser.com.au/frequently-asked-questions.htm

Fuss, D. (1995). *Identification papers*. New York: Routledge.

FWD (feminists with disabilities) for a way forward. (n.d.). Retrieved from http://disabledfeminists.com/

Gailey, E.A. (2007). Self-made women: Cosmetic surgery shows and the construction of female psychopathology. In D. Heller (Ed.), *Makeover television: Realities remodelled* (pp. 107-118). New York: I.B.Tauris.

GarySharp. (2012). Re: The Voice Australia: Darren v Brett [Online forum comment]. Retrieved from http://www.youtube.com/all_comments?threaded=1&v=E0PZuDbLY6U

Gauntlett, D. (2002). *Media, gender and identity: An introduction*. London: Routledge.

georgiegirl66. (2012, March 13). Re: Selena – Lost 700 grams in 4 weeks outside [Online forum comment]. Retrieved from http://www.community.ten.com.au/community/the_biggest_loser

Gillan, J. (2011). *Television and new media: Must-click TV*. New York: Routledge.

Gingras, J. (2005). The defeat of imagination: Repressive codes governing our media. In S. Moorti & K. Ross (Eds.), Introduction: Gender and the plus-size body. *Feminist Media Studies, 5*(2), 255-257. Retrieved from http://www.tandfonline.com/doi/abs/10.1080/14680770500112368

GLAAD (Gay and Lesbian Alliance Against Defamation). (2013). Where We Are on TV 2012–2013. Retrieved from http://www.glaad.org/files/whereweareontv12.pdf

Glee Forum. (2012). Retrieved from http://www.gleeforum.com/

Glenn. (2011, September 2). Re: Disability on the small screen: What's wrong with this picture? [Web log comment]. Retrieved from http://www.abc.net.au/rampup/articles/2011/09/02/3308488.htm

Godlewski, L. R., & Perse, E. M. (2010). Audience activity and reality television: Identification, online activity, and satisfaction. *Communication Quarterly, 58*(2), 148-169.

Goggin, G., & Newell, C. (2003). Imagining diversity: Disability/Film. *Proceedings of Australian & New Zealand Communication Association (ANZCA) International Designing Communication for Diversity Conference.* Brisbane, Australia: Queensland University of Technology.

GoodOldTalk. (n.d.). Grumpy Old Men and Grumpy Old Women [Online forum]. Retrieved from http://goodoldtalk.com/forum/grumpy-old-men-grumpy-old-women

gooseball. (2009, June 11). Re: 10 Years Younger in 10 Days – TV shows [Online forum comment]. Retrieved from http://forums.whirlpool.net.au/archive/1195197

Gordita. (2009, February 9). Re: Saggy skin [Online forum comment]. Retrieved from http://community.ten.com.au/community/the_biggest_loser

Graham, L. (2011). The product of text and 'other' statements: Discourse analysis and the critical use of Foucault. *Educational Philosophy and Theory, 43*(6), 663-674.

Granade, A. S. (2011). 'So here's us, on the raggedy edge': Exoticism and identification in Joss Whedon's *Firefly*. *Popular Music and Society, 34*(5), 621-637.

Gray, J. (2008). *Television entertainment.* New York: Routledge.

Greenberg, B., Eastin, M., Hofschire, L., Lachlan K., & Brownell, K. (2003). Portrayals of overweight and obese individuals on commercial television. *American Journal of Public Health, 93*(8), 1324-1348.

Grumpier Old Men. (n.d.). Grumpier old men [Online forum]. Retrieved from http://www.grumpieroldmen.co.uk

Gullette, M. M. (1997). *Declining to decline: Cultural combat and the politics of the midlife.* Charlottesville, VA: University Press of Virginia.

Gullette, M. M. (2011). *Agewise: Fighting the new ageism in America.* Chicago: University of Chicago Press.

Hall, S. (1980). Encoding/Decoding. In S. Hall, D. Hobson, A. Lowe & P. Willis (Eds.), *Culture, media, language: Working papers in cultural studies, 1972–79* (pp. 41-49). London: Hutchinson.

Haller, B. (2000). If they limp, they lead? News representations and the hierarchy of disability images. In D. Braithwaite & T. Thompson (Eds.), *Handbook of communication and people with disabilities* (pp. 225-237). Mahwah, NJ: Lawrence Erlbaum.

Haller, B. (2010). *Representing disability in an ableist world: Essays on mass media.* Louisville, KY: Avocado Press.

Hardy, M. (2009, July 2). Kissing off year's most vile show [Online review]. Retrieved from http://www.theage.com.au/news/entertainment/tv--radio/years-most-vile-show/2009/07/01/1246127569460.html

Harmer, W. (2009, May 21). Only as young as your next injection [Online review]. Retrieved from http://www.theage.com.au/articles/2009/05/20/1242498758571.html

Harwood, J. (2007). *Understanding communication and aging: Developing knowledge and awareness*. Thousand Oaks, CA: SAGE.

Healey, T., & Ross, K. (2002). Growing old invisibly: Older viewers talk television. *Media, Culture & Society, 24*(1), 105-120.

Hepworth, M. (2000). *Stories of ageing*. Buckingham, England: Open University Press.

Hevey, D. (1997). Controlling interests. In A. Pointon & C. Davies (Eds.), *Framed: Interrogating disability in the media* (pp. 209-213). London: British Film Institute.

Heyes, C. (2007). *Self-Transformations: Foucault, ethics, and normalized bodies*. Oxford: Oxford University Press.

Himes, S. M., & Thompson, J. K. (2007). Fat stigmatization in television shows and movies: A content analysis. *Obesity, 15*(3), 712-718.

Hodgetts, D., Chamberlain, K., & Bassett, G. (2003). Between television and the audience: Negotiating representations of ageing. *Health, 7*(4), 417-438.

Hoffner, C., & Buchanan, M. (2005). Young adults' wishful identification with television characters: The role of perceived similarity and character attributes. *Media Psychology, 7*(4), 325-351.

Holmes, S. (2010). Dreaming a dream: Susan Boyle and celebrity culture. *The Velvet Light Trap, 65*, 74-76.

Holstein, M., Parks, J. A., & Waymack, M. H. (2011). *Ethics, aging, and society: The critical turn*. New York: Springer Publishing Company.

Huff, J. (2001). A 'Horror of Corpulence': Interrogating bantingism and mid-nineteenth-century fat-phobia. In J. E. Braziel & K. LeBesco (Eds.), *Bodies out of bounds: Fatness and transgression* (pp. 39-59). Berkeley, CA: University of California Press.

Idato, M. (2011). For popularity, go with your gut [Online review]. Retrieved from http://www.theage.com.au/entertainment/tv-and-radio/for-popularity-go-with-your-gut-20110216–1aw1a.html

Imcka28. (2009, December 18). Re: Jake's brother [Online web comment]. Retrieved from http://au.tv.yahoo.com/packed-to-the-rafters/forum

inarastarte. (2009, April 23). Re: Motivation [Online forum comment]. Retrieved from http://community.ten.com.au/community/the_biggest_loser

incywebb. (2012, March 6). Re: Margie [Online forum comment]. Retrieved from http://community.ten.com.au/community/the_biggest_loser

Indiefilmchick. (2010, June 28). Re: Huge mistake [Web log comment]. Retrieved from http://www.bigfatblog.com/huge-mistake

inhershoes. (2009, April 22). Re: Ch 7's '10 Years Younger in 10 Days' [Online forum comment]. Retrieved from http://forums.vogue.com.au/showthread.php?t=329712&page=3

InTheWild. (2010, October 5). Re: Packed to the Rafters [Online forum comment]. Retrieved from http://www.mediaspy.org/forum/index.php?/topic/11623-packed-to-the-rafters/page-51?&

iorarua ®. (2010, August 4). Re: Grumpy Old Women Friday evenings late [Online forum comment]. Retrieved from http://www2b.abc.net.au/tmb/Client/Message.aspx?b=81&m=90369&ps=50&dm=1&pd=3

Isabela Rivas. (2012). Re: The Voice Australia: Rachael v Adam – Over the Rainbow [Online forum comment]. Retrieved from http://www.youtube.com/all_comments?v=ndyyZdqv08U

Jacinta gal. (2012a, March 26). Re: Margie [Online forum comment]. Retrieved from http://community.ten.com.au/community/the_biggest_loser

Jacinta gal. (2012b, April 4). Re: Selena's bombshell [Online forum comment]. Retrieved from http://community.ten.com.au/community/the_biggest_loser

Jackie. (2011, May 5). Re: Vera Review: ITV's drama renaissance continues [Online forum comment]. Retrieved from http://channelhopping.onthebox.com/2011/05/01/vera-review-itvs-drama-renaissance-continues/#comment-80778

Jacquee Storozynski-Toll. (2011, May 9). Re: Vera Review: ITV's drama renaissance continues [Online forum comment]. Retrieved from http://channelhopping.onthebox.com/2011/05/01/vera-review-itvs-drama-renaissance-continues/#comment-81999

janknowles. (2009, September 2). Re: Kristian Schmid [Online forum comment]. Retrieved from http://au.tv.yahoo.com/packed-to-the-rafters/forum

jaque_the_ripper. (2012, May 10). Re: How disabled does one have to be before they are considered 'disabled'? [Online forum comment]. Retrieved from http://www.gleeforum.com/index.php/topic/31175-how-disabled-does-one-have-to-be-before-they-are-considered-disabled/

Jenkins, H. (1992). *Textual poachers: Television fans and participatory culture* (2nd ed.). New York: Routledge.

jeschique. (2009, April 22). Re: Ch 7's '10 years younger in 10 days' [Online forum comment]. Retrieved from http://forums.vogue.com.au

Johnson, D. A. (2008). Managing Mr. Monk: Control and the politics of madness. *Critical Studies in Media Communication, 25*(1), 28-47.

Jones, J. M. (2003). Show your real face: A fan study of the UK *Big Brother* transmissions (2000, 2001, 2002). Investigating the boundaries between notions of consumers and producers of factual television. *New Media & Society, 5*(3), 400-421.

Judochop87. (2012, March 13). Re: The Biggest Loser – 2012 [Online forum comment]. Retrieved from http://forums.whirlpool.net.au/archive/1850856

jules363. (2009, March 16). Re: Packed to the Rafters [Online forum comment]. Retrieved from http://www.essentialkids.com.au/forums/lofiversion/index.php/t642685–50.html

june27. (2012, January 27). Re: The Biggest Loser – 2012 [Online forum comment]. Retrieved from http://forums.whirlpool.net.au/archive/1850856#

jungle0005. (2009, February 23). Re: tbl and eating is it just me? [Online forum comment]. Retrieved from http://community.ten.com.au/community/the_biggest_loser

Jutel, A. (2005). Weighing health: The moral burden of obesity. *Social Semiotics, 15*(2), 113-125.

karol. (2009, April 22). Re: Ch 7's '10 years younger in 10 days' [Online forum comment]. Retrieved from http://forums.vogue.com.au

Kavka, M. (2008). *Reality television, affect and intimacy: Reality matters.* Basingstoke, England: Palgrave Macmillan.

KazbahKaren. (2012, March 9). Re: Selena the actress [Online forum comment]. Retrieved from http://www.community.ten.com.au/community/the_biggest_loser

kaz38178. (2009, December 18). Re: Jake's brother [Online forum comment]. Retrieved from http://au.tv.yahoo.com/packed-to-the-rafters/forum

Kelly, A. (2011, March 1). Review: Hot in Cleveland, Skyliving [Online review]. Retrieved from http://suite101.com/article/review-hot-in-cleveland-skyliving-a354358

Kelly, M. (2010, October 25). Should 'fatties' get a room? (Even on TV?) [Web log post]. Retrieved from http://www.marieclaire.com/sex-love/dating-blog/overweight-couples-on-television

Kennedy, G. (2009, November 12). 'Glee': Defying gravity with heart and soul [Online review]. Retrieved from http://latimesblogs.latimes.com/showtracker/2009/11/glee-defying-gravity-with-heart-and-soul/comments/page/2/

Kessler, E., Rakoczy, K., & Staudinger, U. M. (2004). The portrayal of older people in prime time television series: The match with gerontological evidence. *Ageing & Society, 24*(4), 531-552.

Kimdog. (2009, July 11). Will Drop Dead Diva live up to the hype? [Web log post]. Retrieved from http://www.bigfatblog.com/will-drop-dead-diva-live-hype

klouise. (2011, May 4). Re: Vera Review: ITV's drama renaissance continues [Online forum comment]. Retrieved from http://channelhopping.onthebox.com/2011/05/01/vera-review-itvs-drama-renaissance-continues/#comment-80757

Knox, D. (2009a, August 26). Kristian Schmid on Rafters [Online review]. Retrieved from http://www.tvtonight.com.au/2009/08/kristian-schmid-on-rafters.html

Knox, D. (2009b, April 20). Week 17 ratings [Online ratings review]. Retrieved from http://www.tvtonight.com.au/2009/04/week-17-

Lambert, A. (2010). (Re)Producing country: Mapping multiple Australian spaces. *Space and Culture, 13*(3), 304-314.

lambertjessica. (2009, December 18). Re: Jake's brother [Online forum comment]. Retrieved from http://au.tv.yahoo.com/packed-to-the-rafters/forum

Lauredhel. (2009, October 29). Law & order dignity worth and the medical model of disability [Web log post]. Retrieved from http://disabledfeminists.com/2009/10/29/law-order-dignity-worth-and-the-medical-model-of-disability/

Leahcar, R. (2012). Bionic eye story [Web log post]. Retrieved from http://rachaeleahcar94.tumblr.com/post/36042623844/bionic-eye-story

LeBesco, K. (2006). Disability, gender and difference on *The Sopranos*. *Women's Studies in Communication*, *29*(1), 39-59.

LeeLee. (2009, November 5). Re: And if this keeps up, there won't be any [Web log comment]. Retrieved from http://disabledfeminists.com/2009/11/05/and-if-this-keeps-up-there-wont-be-any/

Lewis, T. (2008). Introduction: Revealing the makeover show. *Continuum: Journal of Media & Cultural Studies*, *22*(4), 441-446.

LEXY. (2010, February 4). Re: New reality show: I'm Hotter Than My Daughter [Online forum comment]. Retrieved from http://www.sodahead.com/entertainment/new-reality-show-im-hotter-than-my-daughter/blog-253001/?q=Hotter%20than%20my%20Daughter%20on%20Sodahead&page=5#comments

Littlejlh. (2009a, February 9). Re: Saggy skin [Online forum comment]. Retrieved from http://community.ten.com.au/community/the_biggest_loser

Littlejlh. (2009b, February 1) Re: TBL Weight loss record, Shannan happy, real weight loss expert unhappy [Online forum comment]. Retrieved from http://community.ten.com.au/community/the_biggest_loser

Livingstone, S. (1999). New media, new audiences? *New Media & Society*, *1*(1), 59-66.

Livingstone, S. (2004). The challenge of changing audiences: Or, what is the researcher to do in the age of the internet? Retrieved from http://eprints.lse.ac.uk/archive/00000412

Livingstone, S. (2005). On the relation between audiences and publics: Why audience and public? Retrieved from http://eprints.lse.ac.uk/archive/00000437

Lloyd, R. (2010, September 20). Television review: 'Mike & Molly' [Online review]. Retrieved from http://articles.latimes.com/2010/sep/20/entertainment/la-et-mike-molly-20100920

Longmore, P. (1987). Screening stereotypes: Images of disabled people in television and motion pictures. In A. Gartner & T. Joe (Eds.), *Images of the disabled, disabling images* (pp. 65-78). New York: Praeger.

Longmore, P. (2003). *Why I burned my book: And other essays on disability*. Philadelphia, PA: Temple University Press.

Lorenzo-Dus, N. (2009). 'You're barking mad, I'm out': Impoliteness and broadcast talk. *Journal of Politeness Research: Language, Behaviour, Culture*, *5*(2), 159-187.

Lorié, Á. F. (2011). Forbidden fruit or conventional apple pie? A look at *Sex and the City's* reversal of the female gender. *Media, Culture & Society, 33*(1), 35-51.

Lotz, A. D. (2007). *The television will be revolutionized.* New York: New York University Press.

lozz. (2009, May 14). Re: Ch 7's '10 years younger in 10 days' [Online forum comment]. Retrieved from http://forums.vogue.com.au

Luther, C. A., Ringer Lepre, C. R., & Clark, N. (2012). *Diversity in U.S. mass media.* Chichester, England: Wiley-Blackwell.

MagickalGoddess. (2009, April 23). Re: Ch 7's '10 years younger in 10 days' [Online forum comment]. Retrieved from http://forums.vogue.com.au

Major, B., Spencer, S., Schmader, T., Wolfe, C., & Crocker, J. (1998). Coping with negative stereotypes about intellectual performance: The role of psychological disengagement. *Personality and Social Psychology Bulletin, 24*(1), 34-50.

Mangan, L. (2010, February 23). Cable girl: Hotter Than My Daughter clinging to your last shreds of hope for humanity? BBC3's latest offering should finish you off [Online review]. Retrieved from http://www.guardian.co.uk/tv-and-radio/2010/feb/23/hotter-than-my-daughter-bbc3

Mangan, L. (2012, July 4). TV review: When I get older; River cottage: Three go mad [Online review]. Retrieved from http://www.guardian.co.uk/tv-and-radio/2012/jul/04/when-i-get-older-review

Maria. (2004, November 29). Re: Fat on Reality TV [Web log comment]. Retrieved from http://www.bigfatblog.com/node/842.

Maria-TheGourmetChallenge. (2009, April 22). Re: Ch 7's '10 years younger in 10 days' [Online forum comment]. Retrieved from http://forums.vogue.com.au

MarilynW. (2009, July 11). Re: Will Drop Dead Diva live up to the hype? [Web log comment]. Retrieved from http://www.bigfatblog.com/will-drop-dead-diva-live-hype

Mark. (2010, November 1). Re: The British Comedy Guide [Online forum comment]. Retrieved from http://www.comedy.co.uk/forums

McCormick, K. (2011). A champion of the good life. *Link Disability Magazine, 20*(3). Retrieved from http://linkonline.com.au/read/?/p/view/issueID/13

MediaSpy. (n.d.). Retrieved from http://www.mediaspy.org/

MediaSpy. (2009). Packed to the Rafters [Online forum]. Retrieved from http://www.mediaspy.org/forum/index.php?/topic/11623-packed-to-the-rafters/

Medina, J. (2003). Identity trouble: Disidentification and the problem of difference. *Philosophy & Social Criticism, 29*(6), 655-680.

Meg_Bellamy. (2009, April 22). Re: Ch 7's '10 years younger in 10 days' [Online forum comment]. Retrieved from http://forums.vogue.com.au

meltinzone. (2012, April 26). Betty White's Off Their Rockers [Online review]. Retrieved from http://www.imdb.com/title/tt1879713/reviews

Michael Wenthold. (2011, January 10). Re: Should 'fatties' get a room? (Even on TV?) [Web log comment]. Retrieved from http://www.marieclaire.com/sex-love/dating-blog/overweight-couples-on-television

Miller, T. (2008). The new world makeover. *Continuum: Journal of Media & Cultural Studies, 22*(4), 585-590.

Miss CTree. (2010, November 16). Re: The British Comedy Guide [Online forum comment]. Retrieved from http://www.comedy.co.uk/forums

MissFlick. (2009, April 22). Re: Ch 7's '10 years younger in 10 days' [Online forum comment]. Retrieved from http://forums.vogue.com.au

missmelba. (2009, April 22) Re: Ch 7's '10 years younger in 10 days' [Online forum comment]. Retrieved from http://forums.vogue.com.au

Mitchell, D., & Snyder, S. (2000). *Narrative prosthesis: Disability and the dependencies of discourse.* Ann Arbor, MI: The University of Michigan Press.

Mosher, J. (2001). Setting free the bears: Refiguring fat men on television. In J. E. Braziel & K. LeBesco (Eds.), *Bodies out of bounds: Fatness and transgression* (pp. 166-193). Berkeley, CA: University of California Press.

mrmister. (2012, January 23). Re: The Biggest Loser – 2012 [Online forum comment]. Retrieved from http://forums.whirlpool.net.au/archive/1850856#

MrsLovett1979. (2010, November 9). Re: Sitcoms and other yukky stuff; Mike & Molly [Online forum comment]. Retrieved from http://forums.televisionwithoutpity.com/index.php?showtopic=3198677&st=150

mugclass. (2011, May 3). Re: TV Review: Vera and Exile [Online forum comment]. Retrieved from http://www.guardian.co.uk/tv-and-radio/2011/may/01/tv-review-vera-exile#comment-10573237

Mummery, J., & Rodan, D. (2011). Chewing the communal cud: Community deliberation in broadsheet letters and political blogs. In J. Yearwood & A. Stranieri (Eds.), *Technologies for supporting reasoning communities and collaborative decision making: Cooperative approaches* (pp. 296-318). Hershey, PA: Information Science Reference.

Murphett, A. (2012). New rule: Great voices never get old [Online review]. Retrieved from http://www.theage.com.au/entertainment/tv-and-radio/new-rule-great-voices-never-get-old-20120403–1w9ai.html

Murray, S. (2005a). Introduction to 'Thinking Fat' [Special Issue]. *Social Semiotics, 15*(2), 111-112.

Murray, S. (2005b). (Un/be)coming out? Rethinking fat politics [Special Issue]. *Social Semiotics, 15*(2), 153-163.

Murray, S. (2007). Corporeal knowledges and deviant bodies: Perceiving the fat body. *Social Semiotics, 17*(3), 361-373.

My Milk Spilt. (2011). I am not your cautionary tale [Web log post]. Retrieved from http://mymilkspilt.wordpress.com/2011/02/01/i-am-not-your-cautionary-tale/

~nareen~. (2009, April 22). Re: Ch 7's '10 years younger in 10 days' [Online forum comment]. Retrieved from http://forums.vogue.com.au

Nelson, J. (2000). The media role in building the disability community. *Journal of Mass Media Ethics, 15*(3), 180-193.

nescafed. (2009, April 23). Re: Ch 7's '10 years younger in 10 days' [Online forum comment]. Retrieved from http://forums.vogue.com.au

Newcomb, H., & Hirsch, P. (1994). Television as a cultural forum. In H. Newcomb (Ed.), *Television: The critical view* (5th ed., pp. 503-515). New York: Oxford University Press.

ngayonatkailanman. (2009, 13 April). Re: Susan Boyle singing 'I Dreamed a Dream' from Les Misérables [Online forum comment]. Retrieved from http://www.susan-boyle.com/messages/view/bckzxryvbfymd8qt

nickeroo. (2009, January 24). Re: Are we all sadistic sickos? [Online forum comment]. Retrieved from http://community.ten.com.au/community/the_biggest_loser

Norden, M. (1994). *Cinema of isolation: A history of physical disability in the movies.* New Brunswick, NJ: Rutgers University Press.

NotWithOutAFight. (2010, February 4). Re: New reality show: I'm Hotter Than My Daughter [Online forum comment]. Retrieved from http://www.sodahead.com/entertainment/new-reality-show-im-hotter-than-my-daughter/blog-253001/?q=Hotter%20than%20my%20Daughter%20on%20Sodahead&page=5#comments

NYU Student. (2010, October 28). Re: Marie Claire's size-ism controversy [Online forum comment]. Retrieved from http://www.salon.com/2010/10/27/marie_claire_sizeist_jerk/

O'Hara, L. (2008, July 23). Fat acceptance. *The Drum Opinion* [Web log post]. Retrieved from http://www.abc.net.au/unleashed/32464.html

Oliver, M. (1990, July). *The individual and social models of disability.* Paper presented at the Joint Workshop of the Living Options Group and the Research Unit of the Royal College of Physicians on People with Established Locomotor Disabilities in Hospitals, Leeds, England. Retrieved from http://disability-studies.leeds.ac.uk/files/library/Oliver-in-soc-dis.pdf.

Ouellette, L., & Hay, J. (2008). Makeover television, governmentality and the good citizen. *Continuum: Journal of Media & Cultural Studies, 22*(4), 471-484.

Owen, D. (2010, May 18). GLEE 1.18 – 'Laryngitis' [Web log post]. Retrieved from http://danowen.blogspot.com/2010/05/glee-118-laryngitis.html

OzTAM. (2009). Top 20 programs – Ranking report (E). Retrieved from http://www.oztam.com.au/Archives.aspx?Year=2009

Pandora878. (2009, July 29). Re: Kristian Schmid [Online forum comment]. Retrieved from http://au.tv.yahoo.com/packed-to-the-rafters/forum

pani113. (2009, July 12). Re: Will Drop Dead Diva live up to the hype? [Web log comment]. Retrieved from http://www.bigfatblog.com/will-drop-dead-diva-live-hype

Patch, N. (2012, December 27). Autism in pop culture: Characters on autism spectrum on TV, but do they get it right? [Online review]. Retrieved from http://www.huffingtonpost.ca/2012/12/27/autism-in-pop-culture_n_2369681.html

paul. (2004, November 27). Fat on Reality TV [Web log post]. Retrieved from http://www.bigfatblog.com/node/842.

pawlini. (2009, July 29). Re: Packed to the Rafters [Online forum comment]. Retrieved from http://www.mediaspy.org/forum/index.php?/topic/11623-packed-to-the-rafters/page-35

Pew Research Centre. (2009). *Growing old in America: Expectations vs. reality*. Retrieved from http://www.pewsocialtrends.org/2009/06/29/growing-old-in-america-expectations-vs-reality/

Philo, G., Secker, J., Platt, S., Hendersen, L., McLaughlin, G., & Burnside, J. (1994). The impact of the mass media on public images of mental illness: Media content and audience belief. *Health Education Journal, 53*, 271-281.

pink lipgloss. (2009, April 23). Re: Ch 7's '10 years younger in 10 days' [Online forum comment]. Retrieved from http://forums.vogue.com.au

pttrfan01. (2009, July 29). Re: Kristian Schmid [Online forum comment]. Retrieved from http://au.tv.yahoo.com/packed-to-the-rafters/forum

QitelRemel. (2004, October 1). Re: NBC's The Biggest Loser [Web log comment]. Retrieved from http://www.bigfatblog.com/node/805

Quinlan, M. M., & Bates, B. R. (2008). Dances and discourses of (dis)ability: Heather Mills's embodiment of disability on dancing with the stars. *Text and Performance Quarterly, 28*(1-2), 64-80.

Racer25. (2009, November 29). Re: Packed to the Rafters [Online forum comment]. Retrieved from http://www.mediaspy.org/forum/index.php?/topic/11623-packed-to-the-rafters/page-45

Rayner, P., Wall, P., & Kruger, S. (2004). *AS media studies: The essential introduction* (2nd ed.). London: Routledge.

Redden, G. (2007). Makeover morality and consumer culture. In D. A. Heller (Ed.), *Makeover television: Realities remodelled* (pp. 150-164). London: I. B. Tauris.

Redden, G. (2008). Economy and reflexivity in makeover television. *Continuum: Journal of Media & Cultural Studies, 22*(4), 485-494.

Revera Inc., and the International Federation on Ageing. (2012). *Revera Report on Happiness*. Retrieved from http://www.ageismore.com/Ageismore/Research.aspx

Richards, F. (1908). Billy Bunter. *The magnet*. London: Amalgamated Press.

Richardson, J. E. (2007). *Analysing newspapers: An approach from critical discourse analysis*. Basingstoke, England: Palgrave Macmillan.

Richardson, N. (2010). *Transgressive bodies: Representations in film and popular culture.* Farnham, Surrey: Ashgate Publishing.

Ringrose, J., & Walkerdine, V. (2008). Regulating the abject: The TV make-over as site of neo-liberal reinvention toward bourgeois femininity. *Feminist Media Studies, 8*(3), 227-246.

robyndaustin. (2009, September 12). Re: Jake's brother [Online forum comment]. Retrieved from http://au.tv.yahoo.com/packed-to-the-rafters/forum

Rodan, D., & Balnaves, M. (2010). Media activist websites: The nature of e-participation spaces. *Australian Journalism Review, 32*(1), 27-39.

roe. (2009, April 22). Re: Ch 7's '10 years younger in 10 days' [Online forum comment]. Retrieved from http://forums.vogue.com.au

Rosemary. (2011, April 28). Re: 'I am Cerebral Palsy' – by Erin Gough [Web log comment]. Retrieved from http://walkingisoverrated.com/2008/12/17/i-am-cerebral-palsy-by-erin-gough/

Ross, K. (1997). But where's me in it? Disability, broadcasting and the audience. *Media, Culture & Society, 19*(4), 669-677.

Ross, K., & Moorti, S. (2005). Commentary and criticism is fat still a feminist issue? Gender and the plus size body. *Feminist Media Studies, 5*(1), 83-104.

Ross, S. (2009). *Beyond the box: Television and the internet.* Hoboken, NJ: Whiley-Blackwell.

ryaneco. (2010, November 1). Re: Packed to the Rafters [Online forum comment]. Retrieved from http://www.mediaspy.org/forum/index.php?/topic/11623-packed-to-the-rafters/page-56

Santer, V. (2009). Magazine interview: Vanessa Santer talks with Kristian Schmid about his role on Packed to the Rafters [Online review]. Retrieved from http://kristianschmid.tripod.com/id10.html

Sarah. (2009, September 4). Re: I have another confession … [Web log comment]. Retrieved from http://thinkingofstartingablog.blogspot.com.au/2009/09/i-have-another-confession.html

Selena – Lost 700 grams in 4 weeks outside. (2012, March 12–17). [Online forum thread]. Retrieved from http://www.community.ten.com.au/community/the_biggest_loser

Selena's Bombshell. (2012, April 1–7). [Online forum thread]. Retrieved from http://www.community.ten.com.au/community/the_biggest_loser

Selena the Actress. (2012, March 8–12). [Online forum thread]. Retrieved from http://www.community.ten.com.au/community/the_biggest_loser

Sender, K. (2012). *The makeover: Reality television and reflexive audiences.* New York: New York University Press.

Sender, K., & Sullivan, M. (2008). Epidemics of will, failures of self-esteem: Responding to fat bodies in 'The biggest loser' and 'What not to wear'. *Continuum: Journal of Media & Cultural Studies, 22*(4), 573-584.

Seniors.gov.au. (n.d.). Retrieved from Seniors.gov.au

s.e.smith. (2009, November 12). The transcontinental disability choir: Glee-ful appropriation [Web log post]. Retrieved from http://bitchmagazine.org/post/glee-ful-appropriation

s.e.smith. (2010, February 18). Why I am not riled about every instance of crip drag [Web log post]. Retrieved from http://disabledfeminists.com/2010/02/18/why-i-am-not-riled-about-every-instance-of-crip-drag/

s.e.smith. (2012, June 21). Grey's Anatomy and casual ableism [Web log post]. Retrieved from http://meloukhia.net/2012/06/greys_anatomy_and_casual_ableism.html

Shakespeare, T. (1994). Cultural representation of disabled people: Dustbins for disavowal? *Disability & Society, 9*(3), 283-299.

Shakespeare, T. (1997). Soaps: The story so far. In A. Pointon & C. Davies (Eds.), *Framed: Interrogating disability in the media* (pp. 73-78). London: British Film Institute.

Shakespeare, T. (1999). Art and lies? Representations of disability on film. In M. Corker & S. French (Eds.), *Disability discourse* (pp. 164-172). Buckingham: Open University Press.

Sheppard, A. (2011). Rockin' and rollin' on Fox's *Glee. Disability Studies Quarterly, 31*(1) [Online film review]. Retrieved from http://dsq-sds.org/article/view/1354/1474

Shiny. (2009, April 24). Re: Ch 7's '10 years younger in 10 days' [Online forum comment]. Retrieved from http://forums.vogue.com.au

Siebers, T. (2002). Tender organs, narcissism, and identity politics. In S. Snyder, B. J. Brueggemann & R. Garland-Thomson (Eds.), *Disability studies: Enabling the humanities* (pp. 40-55). New York: The Modern Language Association of America.

Signorielli, N. (2001). Aging on television: The picture in the nineties. *Generations, 25*(3), 34-38.

Signorielli, N. (2004). Aging on television: Messages relating to gender, race, and occupation in prime time. *Journal of Broadcasting & Electronic Media, 48*(2), 279-301.

simple.blossom. (2009). Re: Kristian Schmid [Online forum comment]. Retrieved from http://au.tv.yahoo.com/packed-to-the-rafters/forum

Skeggs, B., & Wood, H. (2008). The labour of transformation and circuits of value 'around' reality television. *Continuum: Journal of Media & Cultural Studies, 22*(4), 559-572.

Skeggs, B., & Wood, H. (2012). *Reacting to reality television: Performance, audience and value.* London: Routledge.

Smith, O. (2005). Shifting Apollo's frame: Challenging the body aesthetic in theater dance. In C. Sandhal & P. Auslander (Eds.), *Bodies in commotion: Disability and performance* (pp. 73-85). Ann Arbor, MI: The University of Michigan Press.

snowbunny54. (2010, October 30). Re: Sitcoms and other yukky stuff; Mike & Molly [Online forum comment]. Retrieved from http://forums.televisionwithoutpity.com/index.php?showtopic=3198677&st=120

Snyder, S., & Mitchell, D. (2006). *Cultural locations of disability*. Chicago: The University of Chicago Press.

Snyder, S., & Mitchell, D. (2010). Body genres: An anatomy of disability in film. In S. Chivers & N. Markotić (Eds.), *The problem body: Projecting disability on film* (pp. 179-206). Columbus, OH: The Ohio State University Press.

Son of Furious. (2010, April 2). Re: New reality show: I'm Hotter Than My Daughter [Online forum comment]. Retrieved from http://www.sodahead.com/entertainment/new-reality-show-im-hotter-than-my-daughter/blog-253001/?q=Hotter%20than%20my%20Daughter%20on%20Sodahead&page=6#comments

Space Crip. (2012, July 23). Twin peaks: Manufacturing quirkiness … and danger [Web log post]. Retrieved from http://spacecrip.wordpress.com/2012/07/23/twin-peaks-manufacturing-quirkiness-and-danger/

Stillyanos. (2012, April 2). Re: Selena's bombshell [Online forum comment]. Retrieved from http://www.community.ten.com.au/community/the_biggest_loser

storm-boy. (2009, February 19). Re: Degrading and wrong [Online forum comment]. Retrieved from http://community.ten.com.au/community/the_biggest_loser

sub101. (2009, February 26). Re: tbl and eating is it just me? [Online forum comment]. Retrieved from http://community.ten.com.au/community/the_biggest_loser

Tang, L., & Yang, P. (2011). Symbolic power and the internet: The power of a 'horse'. *Media, Culture & Society, 33*(5), 675-691.

Television Without Pity. (n.d.). Retrieved from http://www.televisionwithoutpity.com

Terrible Palsy. (2009, September 3). Stereotypes [Web log post]. Retrieved from http://www.terriblepalsy.com/?s=packed+to+the+rafters

The Biggest Loser. (n.d.). Retrieved from http://thebiggestloser.com.au/community.ten.com.au

TheChamp. (2012, July 4). Re: Is the BBC serving older viewers properly? [Web log comment]. Retrieved from http://www.guardian.co.uk/tv-and-radio/tvandradioblog/2012/jul/04/when-i-get-older-bbc

TheDanaCrew. (2009, January 23). Re: Are we all sadistic sickos? [Online forum comment]. Retrieved from http://community.ten.com.au/community/the_biggest_loser

The Drum Opinion. (2008). Re: Fat acceptance [Web log comment]. Retrieved from http://www.abc.net.au/unleashed/32464.html

The Goldfish. (2007). Blogging brings more of us to the table. *Disability Studies Quarterly, 27*(1-2). Retrieved from http://www.dsq-sds.org/article/view/4/4.

TheLoneOutsider. (2011, May 4). Re: Hughes shocks judges with MasterChef refusal [Online forum comment]. Retrieved from http://www.theage.com.au/entertainment/tv-and-radio/hughes-shocks-judges-with-masterchef-refusal-20110504–1e7dt.html#comments

The Songbird. (2012, April 3). Re: Selena's bombshell [Online forum comment]. Retrieved from http://community.ten.com.au/community/the_biggest_loser

Thinking of Starting a Blog. (2009). I have another confession [Web log post and comments]. Retrieved from http://thinkingofstartingablog.blogspot.com.au/2009/09/i-have-another-confession.html

Thoman, E. (1987). How well does television handle social issues? *Media & Values*. Retrieved from http://www.medialit.org/reading-room/how-well-does-television-handle-social-issues

Thomas, L. (2009, February 23). One-armed presenter is scaring children, parents tell BBC [Online review]. Retrieved from http://www.dailymail.co.uk/news/article-1152466/One-armed-presenter-scaring-children-parents-tell-BBC.html

Tim Walker. (2010, October 31). Re: The British Comedy Guide [Online forum comment]. Retrieved from http://www.comedy.co.uk/forums

Too light to be contestants. (2009). [Online forum comment]. Retrieved from http://community.ten.com.au/community/the_biggest_loser

Tuchman, G. (1978). Introduction: The symbolic annihilation of women by the mass media. In G. Tuchman, A. Kaplan Daniels & J. Benét (Eds.), *Hearth and home: Images of women in the mass media* (pp. 3-50). New York: Oxford University Press.

Turner, G. (2009). *Ordinary people and the media: The demotic turn*. London: SAGE.

turtleslittle. (2009). Re: Kristian Schmid [Online forum comment]. Retrieved from http://au.tv.yahoo.com/packed-to-the-rafters/forum

TV.com. (n.d.). Retrieved from http://www.tv.com/

unquisite. (2009, April 22). Re: Ch 7's '10 years younger in 10 days' [Online forum comment]. Retrieved from http://forums.vogue.com.au

Valentine, G., & Sporton, D. (2009). 'How other people see you, it's like nothing that's inside': The impact of processes of disidentification and disavowal on young people's subjectivities. *Sociology, 43*(4), 735-751.

vastmuse. (2012, March 13). Re: The Biggest Loser – 2012 [Online forum comment]. Retrieved from http://forums.whirlpool.net.au/archive/1850856

Vernon, J. A., Williams, J. A., Phillips, T., & Wilson, J. (1991). Media stereotyping: A comparison of the way elderly women and men are portrayed on prime-time television. *Journal of Women & Aging, 2*(4), 55-68.

Vesperi, M. (1985). *City of green benches: Growing old in a new downtown*. Ithaca: Cornell University Press.

Ward, S., O'Regan, T., & Goldsmith, B. (2010). 'Neighbours' to 'Packed to the Rafters': Accounting for longevity in the evolution of Aussie soaps. *Media International Australia, Incorporating Culture & Policy, 136*, 162-176.

Webb, J. (2009). *Understanding representation*. London: SAGE.

Wendell, S. (1996). *The rejected body: Feminist philosophical reflections on disability*. New York: Routledge.

Westender. (2009, July 4). Re: 10 Years Younger in 10 Days [Online forum comment]. Retrieved from http://forums.whirlpool.net.au/archive/1195197

wheelchair dancer. (2009, November 13). Glee [Web log post]. Retrieved from http://cripwheels.blogspot.com.au/2009/11/glee.html

Whirlpool Forum. (2012). The Biggest Loser [Online forum]. Retrieved from http://forums.whirlpool.net.au/archive/1850856

Wilkinson, J.A., and Ferraro, K.F. (2004). Thirty years of ageism research. In Todd D. Nelson (Ed.), *Ageism: Stereotyping and prejudice against older persons* (pp. 339-358). Cambridge, MA: The MIT Press.

Williams, B. T. (2009). *Shimmering literacies: Popular culture and reading and writing online*. New York: Peter Lang.

Williams, R. (1974). *Television: Technology and cultural form*. London: Fontana.

Williams, Z. (2011, May 1). TV Review: Vera and Exile [Online review]. Retrieved from http://www.guardian.co.uk/tv-and-radio/2011/may/01/tv-review-vera-exile

withoutscene. (2009, July 11). Re: Will Drop Dead Diva live up to the hype? [Web log comment]. Retrieved from http://www.bigfatblog.com/will-drop-dead-diva-live-hype

withoutscene. (2010, August 12). A little relief – Savannah Dooley on Camp Shane [Web log post]. Retrieved from http://www.bigfatblog.com/little-relief-savannah-dooley-camp-shane

wleesa. (2009, 18 December). Re: Kristian Schmid [Web log comment]. Retrieved from http://au.tv.yahoo.com/packed-to-the-rafters/forum

Wolf, N. (2002). *The beauty myth: How images of beauty are used against women*. New York: HarperCollins.

Wood, H., & Skeggs, B. (2008). Spectacular mortality: 'Reality' television, individualisation and the remaking of the working class. In D. Hesmondhalgh & J. Toynbee (Eds.), *The media and social theory* (pp. 177-193). London: Routledge.

Woodward, K. (1991). *Aging and its discontents: Freud and other fictions*. Bloomington: Indiana University Press.

Woodward, K. (1999). Introduction. In K. Woodward (Ed.), *Figuring age: Women, bodies, generations* (pp. ix-xxix). Bloomington: Indiana University Press.

workingout. (2009, April 23). Re: Motivation [Online forum comment]. Retrieved from http://community.ten.com.au/community/the_biggest_loser

WORMGERM. (2012, February 28). Re: The Biggest Loser – 2012 [Online forum comment]. Retrieved from http://forums.whirlpool.net.au/archive/1850856

Wout Thielemans. (2011, June 30). Re: The British Comedy Guide [Online forum comment]. Retrieved from http://www.comedy.co.uk/forums

Zoel. (2010, February 4). Re: New reality show: I'm Hotter Than My Daughter [Online forum comment]. Retrieved from http://www.sodahead.com/entertainment/new-reality-show-im-hotter-than-my-daughter/blog-253001/?q=Hotter%20than%20my%20Daughter%20on%20Sodahead&link=ibaf&page=5#comments

Zola, I. (1985). Depictions of disability – metaphor, message and medium in the media: A research and political agenda. *Social Science Journal, 22*(4), 5-17.

Television – Selected References

10 Years Younger (UK, 2004-) Television Makeover Series
10 Years Younger in 10 Days (Australia, 2009) Television Makeover Series
A Fish Called Wanda (1988) dir: Charles Crichton
Absolutely Fabulous (1992-) Television Series
America in Primetime (2011) Television Documentary
As Time Goes By (1992–2005) Television Series
Betty White's Off Their Rockers (2012-) Television Series
Beverly Hills 90210 (1990–2000) Television Series
Billy Bunter of Greyfriars School (1952–1961) Television Series
Boston Legal (2004–2008) Television Series
Brand New You (UK, 2005-) Television Makeover Series
Breaking Bad (2008–2013) Television Series
Britain's Got Talent (2007-) Television Reality Series
Britain's Missing Top Model (2008) Television Reality Series
Carnivàle (2003–2005) Television Series
Cheers (1982–1993) Television Series
Cougar Town (2009-) Television Series
Dallas (1978–1991) Television Series
Dance Your Ass Off (2009–2010) Television Reality Series
Desperate Housewives (2004–2012) Television Series
Embarrassing Fat Bodies (2007-) Television Documentary
Everybody Loves Raymond (1996–2005) Television Series
Extreme Makeover (2002–2007) Television Makeover Series
Extreme Makeover: Weight Loss Edition (2011-) Television Makeover Series
Fat Actress (2005) Television Series
Fat and Fatter (2011–2012) Television Documentary
Fat Camp (2006) Television Documentary
Friday Night Lights (2006–2011) Television Series
Fringe (2008-) Television Series

Getting On (2009–2012) Television Series
Gilmore Girls (2000–2007) Television Series
Glee (2009-) Television Series
Golden Oldies (2012) Television Documentary
Grey's Anatomy (2005-) Television Series
Grumpy Old Men (2003–2006) Television Documentary
Grumpy Old Women (2005–2007) Television Documentary
Harry's Law (2011–2012) Television Series
Home and Away (1988-) Television Series
Hot in Cleveland (2010-) Television Series
Hotter Than My Daughter (2010-) Television Makeover Series
I Want a Famous Face (2004–2005) Television Makeover Series
Jamie's Ministry of Food (UK, 2008) Television Reality Series
Lost (2004–2010) Television Series
MasterChef (Australia, 2009-) Television Reality Series
Mike & Molly (2010-) Television Series
My Big Fat Fetish (2013) Television Documentary Series
My Generation (2008) Television Documentary Series
NCIS (2003-) Television Series
Neighbours (1985-) Television Series
New Tricks (2003-) Television Series
Nip/Tuck (2003–2010) Television Series
One Foot in the Grave (1990–2000) Television Series
Quads! (2001–2002) Television Series
Packed to the Rafters (2008-) Television Series
Pelswick (2000–2002) Television Series
Sex and the City (1998–2004) Television Series
The Biggest Loser (Australia, 2006-) Television Makeover Series
The Biggest Loser: Couples (Australia, 2009) Television Makeover Series
The Biggest Loser: Singles (Australia, 2012) Television Makeover Series
The Dukes of Hazzard (1979–1985) Television Series
The Golden Girls (1985–1992) Television Series
The King of Queens (1998–2007) Television Series
The Practice (1997–2004) Television Series
The Sopranos (1999–2007) Television Series
The Swan (2004) Television Makeover Series
The Voice (Australia, 2012-) Television Reality Series
The West Wing (1999–2006) Television Series
The Young Ones (1982–1984) Television Series
Twin Peaks (1990–1991) Television Series
Two and a Half Men (2003-) Television Series
Vera (2011-) Television Series

When I Get Older (2012) Television Documentary Series
When Teenage Meets Old Age (2011) Television Documentary Series
Winners & Losers (2011-) Television Series

Index

For Product Safety Concerns and Information please contact our EU
representative GPSR@taylorandfrancis.com
Taylor & Francis Verlag GmbH, Kaufingerstraße 24, 80331 München, Germany

www.ingramcontent.com/pod-product-compliance
Ingram Content Group UK Ltd.
Pitfield, Milton Keynes, MK11 3LW, UK
UKHW011017180926
475701UK00004B/783

* 9 7 8 1 1 3 8 2 5 4 5 9 6 *